The Science-Backed Acid Reflux Diet Cookbook

365 Days of No-Stress and Delicious Recipes to Relieve GERD, Soothe Your Symptoms, Improve Digestion, and Enhance Well-Being | 28-Day Meal Plan & Full Color Pictures Included

DR. STELLA A. GWIN

Copyright Page

TABLE OF CONTENTS

UNDERSTANDING ACID REFLUX

What is Acid Reflux?

Acid reflux, also known as gastroesophageal reflux disease (GERD) when chronic, is a condition in which stomach acid flows back into the esophagus, the tube connecting your throat and stomach. This backflow, or reflux, can cause irritation and inflammation of the esophagus, leading to various uncomfortable symptoms.

When you eat, food passes down the esophagus and into the stomach through a valve called the lower esophageal sphincter (LES). Normally, the LES closes tightly after food enters the stomach. However, if the LES is weak or relaxes inappropriately, stomach acid can seep back into the esophagus, causing the burning sensation known as heartburn.

SYMPTOMS AND TRIGGERS

The most common symptom of acid reflux is heartburn, a burning pain or discomfort that may move from your stomach to your abdomen or chest, and even up into your throat. Other symptoms can include:

- **Regurgitation:** A sour or bitter-tasting acid backing up into your throat or mouth.
- **Dysphagia:** Difficulty swallowing.
- Chronic cough or throat clearing.
- Hoarseness or sore throat.
- A feeling of a lump in the throat.
- Bloating or burping.
- Nausea.

While occasional acid reflux is common and can occur in healthy individuals, frequent or severe symptoms may indicate GERD, which requires medical attention and long-term management.

COMMON TRIGGERS:

Dietary Choices:

- Fatty or Fried Foods: These slow down digestion and keep food in your stomach longer.
- Spicy Foods: Can irritate the esophagus lining.
- Citrus Fruits: High acidity can trigger reflux.
- Tomato-Based Products: Also highly acidic.
- Chocolate: Contains caffeine and theobromine, which can relax the LES.
- Garlic and Onions: Can cause acid reflux in some individuals.
- Carbonated Beverages: Increase stomach pressure and can push acid into the esophagus.
- Alcohol: Relaxes the LES.

Lifestyle Factors:

- Overeating: Eating large meals increases stomach pressure.
- Eating Before Bedtime: Lying down soon after eating can lead to acid reflux.
- Smoking: Weakens the LES and increases acid production.
- Obesity: Excess weight can put pressure on the abdomen, pushing stomach contents into the esophagus.
- Stress: Can increase acid production and cause changes in eating habits that worsen symptoms.

Medical Conditions and Medications:

- Hiatal Hernia: Part of the stomach pushes up through the diaphragm into the chest cavity, disrupting the LES function.
- Pregnancy: Increased pressure on the abdomen and hormonal changes can cause acid reflux.
- Certain Medications: Such as aspirin, ibuprofen, certain muscle relaxers, or blood pressure medications.

THE SCIENCE BEHIND ACID REFLUX

Acid reflux is fundamentally linked to the malfunction of the lower esophageal sphincter (LES). When functioning correctly, the LES acts as a barrier to prevent stomach contents from flowing back into the esophagus. Several factors contribute to LES dysfunction:

- **LES Pressure**: Normally, the LES maintains a higher pressure than the stomach, preventing reflux. If this pressure difference is reduced, reflux can occur. Factors that can lower LES pressure include certain foods, medications, and lifestyle habits.
- **Gastric Emptying:** Delayed gastric emptying, where the stomach takes longer to empty its contents, can increase the risk of acid reflux. Conditions like gastroparesis (slow stomach emptying) are often associated with chronic reflux.
- **Esophageal Motility:** Proper movement and clearance of swallowed food down the esophagus and into the stomach are essential. If esophageal motility is impaired, acid can remain in contact with the esophagus for longer periods, causing damage and symptoms.
- **Hiatal Hernia:** This condition can compromise the normal functioning of the LES by altering the pressure dynamics between the chest and abdomen.

THE ROLE OF INFLAMMATION

Repeated exposure to stomach acid can cause inflammation of the esophageal lining, a condition known as esophagitis. This inflammation can lead to complications such as:

- **Esophageal Strictures:** Narrowing of the esophagus due to scar tissue formation, which can cause swallowing difficulties.

- **Barrett's Esophagus:** A condition where the cells lining the esophagus change due to chronic acid exposure, increasing the risk of esophageal cancer.
- **Esophageal Ulcers:** Open sores in the esophagus that can bleed and cause pain.

Understanding the science and mechanisms behind acid reflux helps in managing the condition more effectively. By identifying and addressing the specific factors that contribute to your symptoms, you can take targeted steps to reduce or eliminate them, improving your quality of life.

ROLE OF DIET IN MANAGING ACID REFLUX

FOODS TO AVOID

Managing acid reflux effectively often begins with dietary changes. Certain foods can exacerbate acid reflux symptoms, and understanding these triggers is crucial for creating a diet that promotes digestive health.

- **High-Fat Foods:** Foods high in fat, such as fried items, fatty cuts of meat, and full-fat dairy products, can relax the lower esophageal sphincter (LES). This relaxation allows stomach acid to escape into the esophagus, causing reflux. Additionally, high-fat foods delay stomach emptying, which increases the likelihood of acid reflux.
  - **Examples to Avoid:** French fries, fried chicken, hamburgers, bacon, cheese, ice cream.
  - **Healthier Alternatives:** Opt for grilled, baked, or steamed foods. Choose lean meats such as chicken breast, turkey, or fish, and low-fat or non-dairy milk options.
- **Spicy Foods:** Spices can irritate the esophagus and trigger reflux symptoms in some people. Capsaicin, the compound that makes chili peppers hot, can slow digestion and increase the risk of heartburn.
  - **Examples to Avoid:** Chili peppers, hot sauce, curry, spicy sausages.
  - **Healthier Alternatives:** Use herbs and mild spices like basil, oregano, ginger, and parsley to add flavor without the burn.
- **Citrus Fruits and Juices:** Citrus fruits are highly acidic and can exacerbate acid reflux symptoms by increasing stomach acid production.
  - **Examples to Avoid:** Oranges, grapefruits, lemons, limes, orange juice.
  - **Healthier Alternatives:** Consider low-acid fruits like bananas, melons, apples, and pears. Non-citrus juices such as apple juice or pear juice are also good options.

- **Tomatoes and Tomato-Based Products:** Tomatoes are acidic and can trigger reflux symptoms. This includes not only fresh tomatoes but also tomato sauce, ketchup, and salsa.
  - **Examples to Avoid:** Tomato sauce, marinara, ketchup, salsa.
  - **Healthier Alternatives:** Use roasted red peppers or basil pesto as a pasta sauce alternative. Experiment with non-tomato-based sauces like béchamel or a simple olive oil and garlic mixture.
- **Chocolate:** Chocolate contains both caffeine and theobromine, which can relax the LES and increase reflux.
  - **Examples to Avoid:** Chocolate bars, chocolate desserts, hot cocoa.
  - **Healthier Alternatives:** Satisfy your sweet tooth with non-citrus fruits or a small amount of dark chocolate with minimal additives. Carob is a caffeine-free alternative that can be used in baking.
- **Garlic and Onions:** These vegetables can cause stomach acid to increase and irritate the esophagus, particularly when consumed raw.
  - **Examples to Avoid:** Raw garlic and onions, garlic bread, onion rings.
  - **Healthier Alternatives:** Cooked onions and garlic may be less likely to cause symptoms, or use mild alternatives like chives and shallots.

- **Caffeinated and Carbonated Beverages:** Caffeine can increase stomach acid production, and carbonation can cause the stomach to expand, pushing stomach contents up into the esophagus.
    - **Examples to Avoid:** Coffee, tea, sodas, energy drinks.
    - **Healthier Alternatives:** Opt for herbal teas like chamomile or ginger tea. Still water and non-citrus infused waters are also good choices.
- **Alcohol:** Alcohol can relax the LES and increase stomach acid production.
    - **Examples to Avoid:** Beer, wine, cocktails.
    - **Healthier Alternatives:** If you choose to drink alcohol, do so in moderation and opt for lower-acid options like light beer or dry white wine. Avoid mixing with citrus juices or other acidic mixers.

FOODS TO INCLUDE

While avoiding trigger foods is essential, incorporating foods that can help manage acid reflux is equally important. These foods can soothe the digestive system, reduce inflammation, and prevent reflux episodes.

1. **Non-Citrus Fruits**: These are less likely to trigger reflux and are generally soothing to the digestive tract.
   - **Examples**: Bananas, melons, apples, pears.
   - **Benefits**: These fruits are low in acid and high in fiber, which can help absorb stomach acid and prevent reflux.
2. **Vegetables**: Most vegetables are low in fat and sugar, making them an excellent choice for managing acid reflux.
   - **Examples**: Leafy greens, broccoli, cauliflower, asparagus, cucumbers.
   - **Benefits**: These vegetables are nutrient-dense and help reduce stomach acid. They also contain fiber, which promotes healthy digestion.
3. **Whole Grains**: High in fiber, whole grains can help absorb stomach acid and reduce the likelihood of reflux.
   - **Examples**: Oatmeal, brown rice, whole wheat bread, quinoa.
   - **Benefits**: Whole grains are filling and can prevent overeating, which is a common trigger for acid reflux.
4. **Lean Proteins**: Low-fat protein sources are less likely to trigger reflux and help maintain muscle mass and overall health.
   - **Examples**: Chicken breast, turkey, fish, tofu, beans.
   - **Benefits**: These proteins are easier to digest and do not promote acid production like high-fat meats.

- **Healthy Fats:** Incorporate healthy fats in moderation, as they are essential for overall health but can also be easier on the digestive system.
    - **Examples:** Avocado, nuts, seeds, olive oil.
    - **Benefits:** Healthy fats can help reduce inflammation and provide essential fatty acids for overall well-being.
- **Herbal Teas:** Certain herbal teas can soothe the digestive system and reduce reflux symptoms.
    - **Examples:** Chamomile tea, ginger tea, licorice root tea.
    - **Benefits:** These teas have anti-inflammatory and soothing properties that can help manage reflux symptoms.

IMPORTANCE OF EATING HABITS AND TIMING

How and when you eat can be just as important as what you eat when managing acid reflux. Adopting healthy eating habits and timing your meals correctly can significantly reduce symptoms.

- **Smaller, More Frequent Meals**: Eating smaller portions more frequently throughout the day can prevent the stomach from becoming too full, which can reduce the risk of acid reflux.
  - **Tip**: Aim for 5-6 small meals or snacks instead of 3 large meals.
- **Chew Thoroughly and Eat Slowly**: Taking your time to chew food thoroughly and eating slowly can improve digestion and reduce the likelihood of reflux.
  - **Tip**: Put down your fork between bites and savor each mouthful.
- **Avoid Eating Close to Bedtime**: Lying down soon after eating can trigger acid reflux. It's best to finish eating at least 2-3 hours before lying down.
  - **Tip**: If you're hungry close to bedtime, opt for a light snack that is easy to digest.
- **Elevate the Head of Your Bed**: If you experience nighttime reflux, elevating the head of your bed by about 6-8 inches can prevent stomach acid from flowing back into the esophagus.
  - **Tip**: Use bed risers or a wedge pillow to keep your upper body elevated.
- **Stay Upright After Eating**: Avoid lying down or reclining for at least 2-3 hours after meals to prevent reflux.
  - **Tip**: Go for a gentle walk after meals to aid digestion.
- **Maintain a Healthy Weight**: Excess weight can put pressure on the abdomen, pushing stomach contents into the esophagus.
  - **Tip**: Incorporate regular physical activity and a balanced diet to achieve and maintain a healthy weight.

- **Hydrate Wisely**: Drink plenty of water throughout the day, but avoid drinking large quantities during meals, which can expand the stomach and increase reflux risk.
    - **Tip**: Sip water between meals and limit beverages during meals.

28-DAY MEAL PLAN

WEEK 1

	BREAKFAST	LUNCH	DINNER
DAY 1	Tropical Oatmeal Smoothie	Romaine and Strawberry Salad	Millet pilaf
DAY 2	Banana Almond Smoothie	Carrot Ginger Soup	Shrimp and Veggie Stir-Fry
DAY 3	Berry Oat Smoothie	Tuna and White Bean Salad	Mango Nice Cream
DAY 4	Peanut Butter Banana Smoothie	Vegetable and Hummus Wrap	Baked Salmon with Quinoa and Asparagus
DAY 5	Ginger Honey Smoothie	Cucumber Salad	Beef and Broccoli
DAY 6	Egg and Veggie Scramble	Lentil and Vegetable Stew	Stuffed Bell Peppers
DAY 7	Sweet Potato Hash	Potato Leek Soup	Chicken and Pesto Pasta

WEEK 2

	BREAKFAST	LUNCH	DINNER
DAY 1	Zucchini Bread	Watermelon and Feta Salad	Grilled Portobello Mushrooms
DAY 2	Boiled Eggs	Butternut Squash Soup	Zoodle Pad Thai
DAY 3	Veggie Egg Muffins	Chicken Kabobs with Bell Peppers	Bulgur Wheat Tabbouleh
DAY 4	Oat Porridge with Pears	Broccoli and Tofu Stir-Fry	Eggplant Parmesan
DAY 5	Cucumber and Tomato Salad	Herb Crusted Haddock	Beef and Broccoli
DAY 6	Tofu Scramble	Turkey Meatloaf	Prawn Cocktail with Avocado
DAY 7	Sweet Potato Hash	Trout Almondine	Chicken and Veggie Kebabs

Repeat Week 1 and Week 2 to complete the 28-Day Meal Plan.
 Each week has a mix of lean proteins, complex carbohydrates, healthy fats, and fiber-rich foods to ensure optimal digestive health.

TROPICAL OATMEAL SMOOTHIE

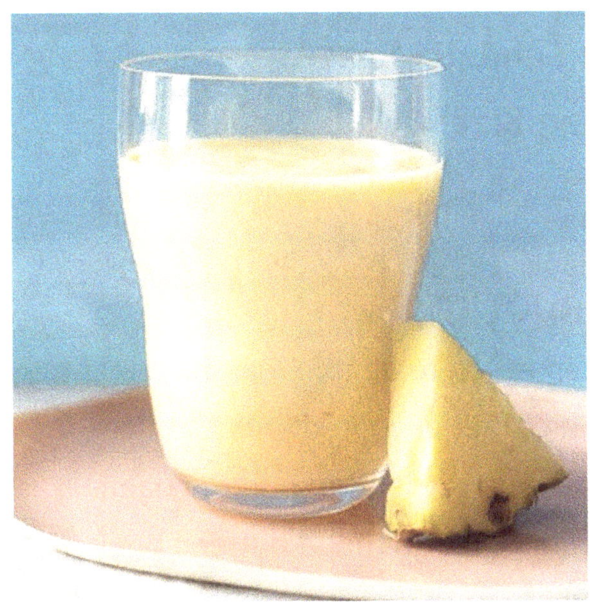

Prep Time: 10 Mins

Serving Size: 2

INGREDIENTS

- 1/2 cup old-fashioned oats
- 1 cup unsweetened almond milk (or other non-dairy milk)
- 1 banana, frozen
- 1/2 cup pineapple chunks, frozen
- 1/2 cup mango chunks, frozen
- 1 tablespoon chia seeds
- 1/2 teaspoon ground ginger
- 1/2 teaspoon ground turmeric
- 1 teaspoon honey (optional)
- 1/2 teaspoon vanilla extract (optional)
- Ice cubes (optional, for a thicker consistency)

NUTRITIONAL FACTS

- Calories: 250kcal | Protein: 5g
- Carbohydrates: 50g | Fiber: 7g
- Sugars: 25g | Fat: 5g

INSTRUCTIONS

- Prepare the Oats: If desired, soak the oats in almond milk for a few hours or overnight to soften them. This step is optional but can make the smoothie creamier.
- Blend the Ingredients: Add the oats, almond milk, frozen banana, pineapple chunks, mango chunks, chia seeds, ground ginger, and ground turmeric to a blender.
- Optional Add-ins: Add honey and vanilla extract if using.
- Blend: Blend until smooth. If the smoothie is too thick, add more almond milk until the desired consistency is reached. For a thicker smoothie, add a few ice cubes and blend again.
- Serve: Pour into two glasses and serve immediately.

BANANA ALMOND SMOOTHIE

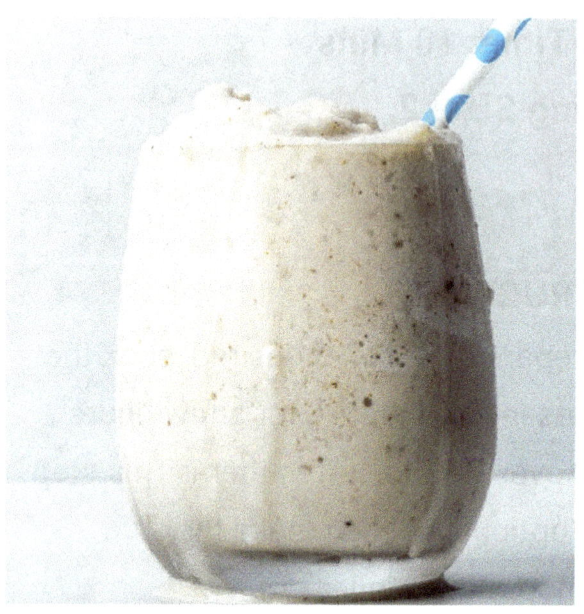

Cook Time: 5 Mins

Serving Size: 1

INSTRUCTIONS

- Prepare Ingredients: Peel the banana and gather all ingredients.
- Combine in Blender: Add the banana, almond milk, almond butter, honey (if using), ground cinnamon, and ice (if using) into a blender.
- Blend: Blend on high until smooth and creamy.
- Serve: Pour into a glass and enjoy immediately.

INGREDIENTS

- 1 ripe banana
- 1 cup almond milk (unsweetened)
- 1 tablespoon almond butter
- 1 teaspoon honey (optional, for sweetness)
- 1/2 teaspoon ground cinnamon
- 1/2 cup ice (optional, for a thicker smoothie)

NUTRITIONAL FACTS

- Calories: 250 kcal
- Total Fat: 11g
- Total Carbohydrates: 36g
- Dietary Fiber: 5g
- Sugars: 19g
- Protein: 5g

BERRY OAT SMOOTHIE

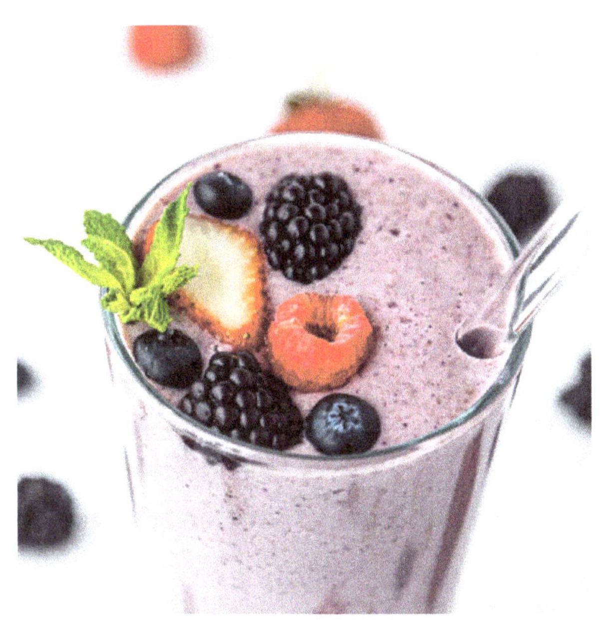

Prep Time: 5 Mins

Serving Size: 1

INGREDIENTS

- 1/2 cup rolled oats
- 1 cup almond milk (unsweetened)
- 1/2 cup frozen blueberries
- 1/2 cup frozen strawberries
- 1/2 banana
- 1 tablespoon chia seeds
- 1/2 teaspoon ground ginger
- 1 teaspoon honey (optional)

NUTRITIONAL FACTS

- Calories: 290kcal
- Protein: 6g
- Carbohydrates: 55g
- Dietary Fiber: 10g
- Sugars: 21g
- Fat: 6g

INSTRUCTIONS

- Prepare the Ingredients: Ensure the oats, fruits, and other ingredients are ready for blending.
- Blend: Add the rolled oats and almond milk to a blender. Blend on high speed for about 30 seconds until the oats are finely ground and mixed with the milk.
- Add Fruits: Add the frozen blueberries, frozen strawberries, banana, chia seeds, and ground ginger to the blender. If desired, add honey for extra sweetness.
- Blend Smooth: Blend all ingredients on high speed for 1-2 minutes until smooth and creamy. If the smoothie is too thick, add a bit more almond milk and blend again.
- Serve: Pour the smoothie into a glass and enjoy immediately.

GINGER HONEY SMOOTHIE

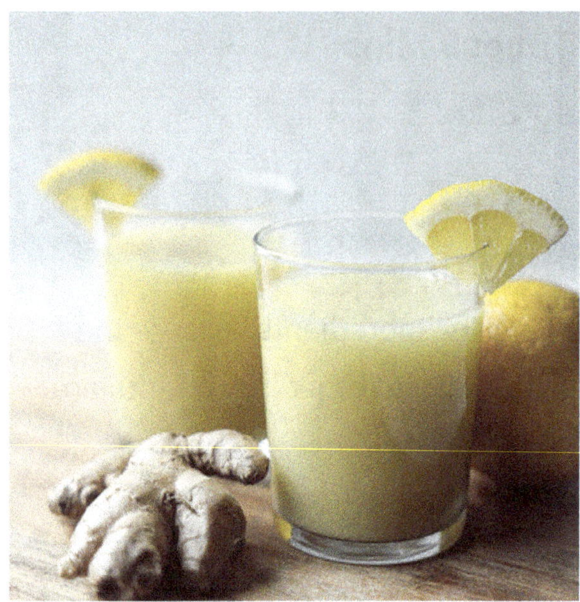

Prep Time: 10 Mins

Serving Size: 2

INSTRUCTIONS

- Peel and grate the fresh ginger.
- Peel and slice the banana, then freeze the slices for at least 2 hours prior to making the smoothie (if not using already frozen banana).
- Measure out all other ingredients.
- In a blender, combine the almond milk, frozen banana, Greek yogurt (if using), grated ginger, honey, ground turmeric, fresh pineapple chunks, vanilla extract, and ice cubes.
- Blend on high speed until smooth and creamy.
- Pour the smoothie into two glasses.
- Enjoy immediately for best taste and texture.

INGREDIENTS

- 1 cup unsweetened almond milk (or any non-dairy milk)
- 1 medium banana, frozen
- 1/2 cup Greek yogurt (optional, can use dairy-free yogurt if preferred)
- 1 tablespoon fresh ginger, grated
- 1 tablespoon honey
- 1/2 teaspoon ground turmeric
- 1/2 cup fresh pineapple chunks (or 100% pineapple juice)
- 1/2 teaspoon vanilla extract
- 1/2 cup ice cubes

NUTRITIONAL FACTS

- Calories: 160 kcal
- Protein: 5g
- Carbohydrates: 32g
- Dietary Fiber: 3g
- Sugars: 22g
- Fat: 2g

WHOLE GRAIN MUFFIN

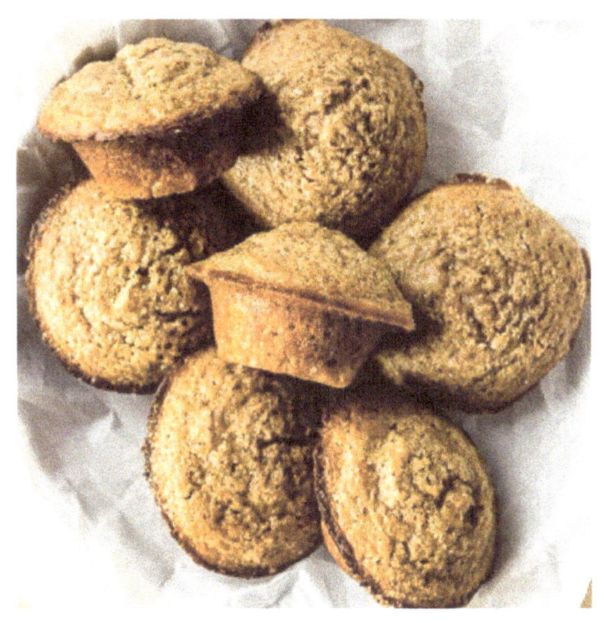

Cook Time: 25 Mins

Serving Size: 12

INGREDIENTS

- 1 ½ cups whole wheat flour
- 1 cup old-fashioned oats
- 1 teaspoon baking soda
- 1 teaspoon baking powder
- ½ teaspoon salt
- 1 teaspoon ground cinnamon
- ½ teaspoon ground ginger
- ½ teaspoon ground nutmeg
- 1 cup unsweetened applesauce
- ½ cup honey or maple syrup
- 2 large eggs, lightly beaten
- ⅓ cup low-fat plain yogurt or Greek yogurt
- ¼ cup unsweetened almond milk or any non-dairy milk
- 1 teaspoon vanilla extract
- 1 medium apple, peeled, cored, and grated (optional)

INSTRUCTIONS

- Preheat your oven to 350°F (175°C). Line a 12-cup muffin tin with paper liners or lightly grease the tin with non-stick cooking spray.
- In a large bowl, combine the whole wheat flour, oats, baking soda, baking powder, salt, cinnamon, ginger, and nutmeg. Mix well to ensure all dry ingredients are evenly distributed.
- In another bowl, whisk together the applesauce, honey (or maple syrup), eggs, yogurt, almond milk, and vanilla extract until well combined.
- Add the wet ingredients to the dry ingredients and stir until just combined. Do not overmix; it's okay if there are a few lumps.
- If using, fold in the grated apple gently into the batter.
- Divide the batter evenly among the 12 muffin cups.

NUTRITIONAL FACTS

- Calories: 150kcal
- Total Fat: 2g
- Carbohydrates: 30g
- Dietary Fiber: 4g
- Sugars: 15g
- Protein: 4g

INSTRUCTIONS

- Bake in the preheated oven for 20-25 minutes, or until a toothpick inserted into the center of a muffin comes out clean.
- Allow the muffins to cool in the tin for 5 minutes before transferring them to a wire rack to cool completely.

AVOCADO TOAST

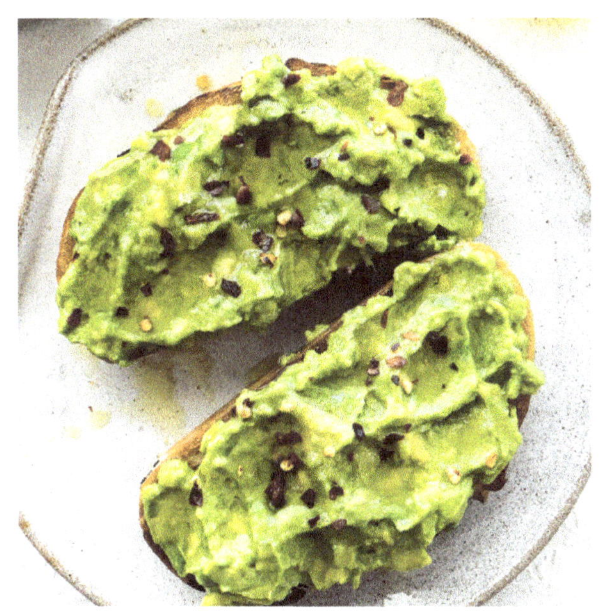

Cook Time: 10 Mins

Serving Size: 1

INGREDIENTS

- 1 slice whole-grain bread (toasted)
- 1/2 ripe avocado
- 1 teaspoon lemon juice (optional, if tolerated)
- Salt to taste (use sparingly)
- Freshly ground black pepper to taste
- 1 tablespoon finely chopped fresh basil

INSTRUCTIONS

- Toast the whole-grain bread until it is golden and crispy.
- While the bread is toasting, scoop the avocado into a bowl and mash it with a fork.
- Add lemon juice, salt, and pepper to the mashed avocado, mixing well.
- Spread the avocado mixture evenly on the toasted bread.
- Sprinkle the chopped basil on top.
- Serve immediately and enjoy.

NUTRITIONAL FACTS

- Calories: 220
- Protein: 4g
- Carbohydrates: 26g
- Dietary Fiber: 8g
- Sugars: 3g
- Total Fat: 13g

EGG WHITE SCRAMBLE

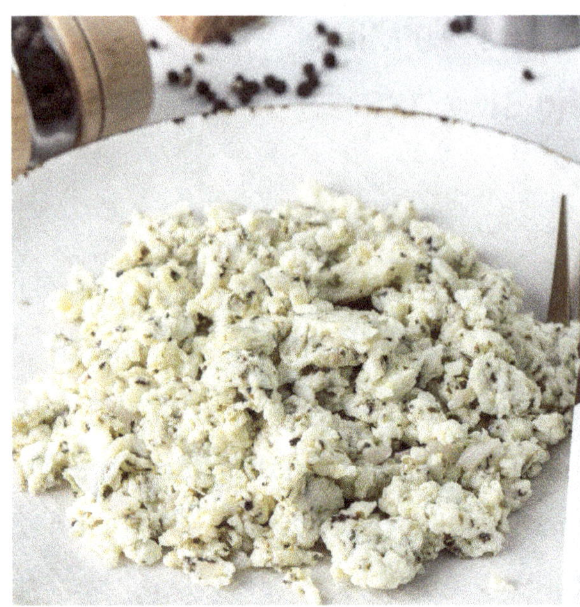

Cook Time: 10

Serving Size: 2

INGREDIENTS

- 6 large egg whites
- 1/4 cup skim milk or unsweetened almond milk
- 1/2 cup spinach, chopped
- 1/2 cup bell peppers (red or green), diced
- 1/4 cup mushrooms, sliced
- 1/4 teaspoon turmeric
- 1/4 teaspoon salt (optional, to taste)
- 1/4 teaspoon black pepper (optional, to taste)
- 1 tablespoon olive oil or a non-stick cooking spray

INSTRUCTIONS

- **Preparation:**
- Whisk egg whites and milk together.
- **Cooking:**
- Heat olive oil or spray a skillet over medium heat.
- Sauté bell peppers and mushrooms for 3-4 minutes.
- Add spinach and cook for 1-2 minutes.
- **Scrambling:**
- Pour egg mixture into the skillet, add turmeric, salt, and pepper.
- Stir gently until eggs are fully cooked, about 3-4 minutes.
- **Serving:**
- Divide onto two plates and serve immediately.

NUTRITIONAL FACTS

- Calories: 110kcal | Protein: 14g
- Carbohydrates: 4g
- Fiber: 1g
- Sugars: 2g
- Fat: 4g

ZUCCHINI BREAD

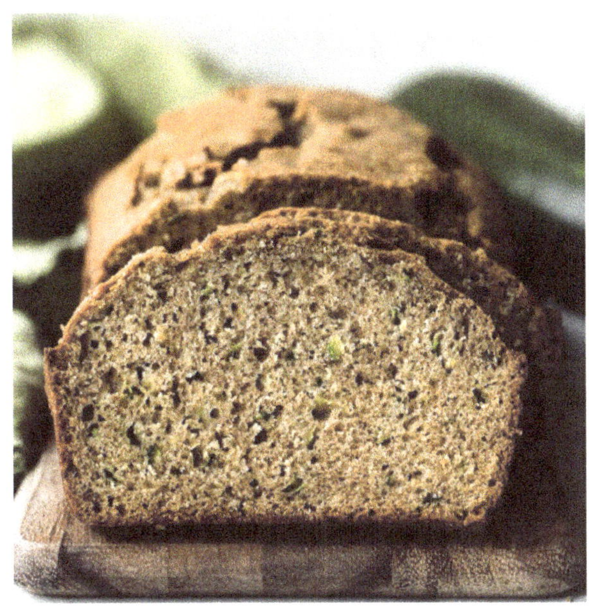

Cook Time: 55 Mins

Serving Size: 12

INGREDIENTS

- 2 cups grated zucchini (about 2 medium zucchinis)
- 1 ½ cups whole wheat flour
- ½ cup all-purpose flour
- 1 tsp baking soda
- 1 tsp baking powder
- ½ tsp salt
- 1 tsp ground cinnamon
- ¼ tsp ground ginger
- ¼ cup olive oil
- ¾ cup unsweetened applesauce
- 2 large eggs
- 1 tsp vanilla extract
- ½ cup honey or maple syrup
- ½ cup chopped walnuts (optional)
- ½ cup raisins or chopped dates (optional)

INSTRUCTIONS

- Preheat oven to 350°F (175°C). Grease or line a 9x5-inch loaf pan.
- Grate zucchini and set aside.
- In a large bowl, whisk flours, baking soda, baking powder, salt, cinnamon, and ginger.
- In another bowl, whisk olive oil, applesauce, eggs, vanilla, and honey or maple syrup.
- Combine wet and dry ingredients, then fold in zucchini, walnuts, and raisins or dates if using.
- Pour batter into loaf pan and bake for 50-55 minutes, until a toothpick comes out clean.
- Cool in pan for 10 minutes, then transfer to a wire rack to cool completely.

NUTRITIONAL FACTS

- Calories: 160kcal | Fat: 6g
- Total Carbohydrates: 24g
- Dietary Fiber: 3g
- Sugars: 10g
- Protein: 3g

BOILED EGGS

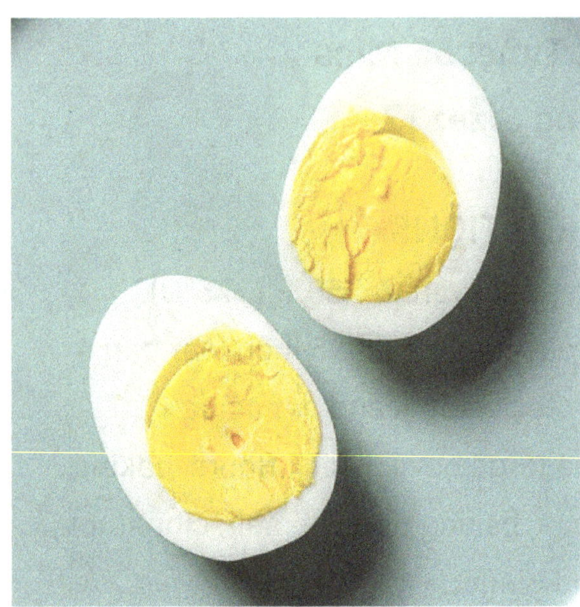

Cook Time: 12 Mins

Serving Size: 2

INGREDIENTS

- 4 large eggs
- Water (enough to cover the eggs in a saucepan)
- Pinch of salt (optional)

NUTRITIONAL FACTS

- Calories: 140kcal
- Protein: 12g
- Fat: 10g
- Carbohydrates: 1g
- Dietary Fiber: 0g
- Sugars: 1g

INSTRUCTIONS

- Place the eggs in a single layer at the bottom of a saucepan. Add enough water to cover the eggs by about an inch.
- Add a pinch of salt to the water (optional, helps prevent cracking). Bring the water to a boil over medium-high heat.
- Once the water reaches a rolling boil, turn off the heat and cover the pan with a lid. Let the eggs sit in the hot water for 9-12 minutes, depending on how well-cooked you like your yolks.
- After the time has elapsed, transfer the eggs to a bowl of ice water to stop the cooking process. Let them cool for at least 5 minutes.
- Gently tap the eggs on a hard surface and peel away the shells. Serve immediately or refrigerate for later use.

OAT PORRIDGE WITH PEARS

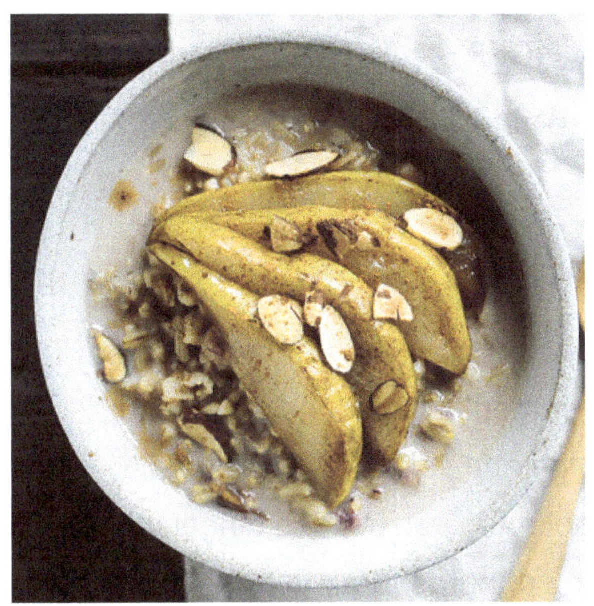

Cook Time: 15 Mins

Serving Size: 2

INGREDIENTS

- 1 cup rolled oats
- 2 cups water or almond milk (unsweetened)
- 1 ripe pear, peeled, cored, and diced
- 1 tablespoon honey (optional, for sweetness)
- 1/2 teaspoon ground cinnamon
- 1/4 teaspoon ground ginger
- A pinch of salt

NUTRITIONAL FACTS

- Calories: 250 kcal
- Carbohydrates: 50g
- Protein: 6g
- Fat: 3g
- Fiber: 7g
- Sugar: 12g

INSTRUCTIONS

- Prepare Ingredients: Peel, core, and dice the pear.
- Cook Oats: In a medium-sized pot, bring the water or almond milk to a boil. Add the rolled oats and reduce the heat to low. Simmer for about 5 minutes, stirring occasionally.
- Add Pear and Spices: Stir in the diced pear, ground cinnamon, ground ginger, and a pinch of salt. Continue to cook for another 5 minutes, or until the oats are tender and the pear is soft.
- Optional Sweetening: If desired, stir in the honey for added sweetness. Mix well to combine.
- Serve: Divide the porridge into two bowls. Let it cool slightly before serving to avoid irritation from hot food.

CARROT GINGER SOUP

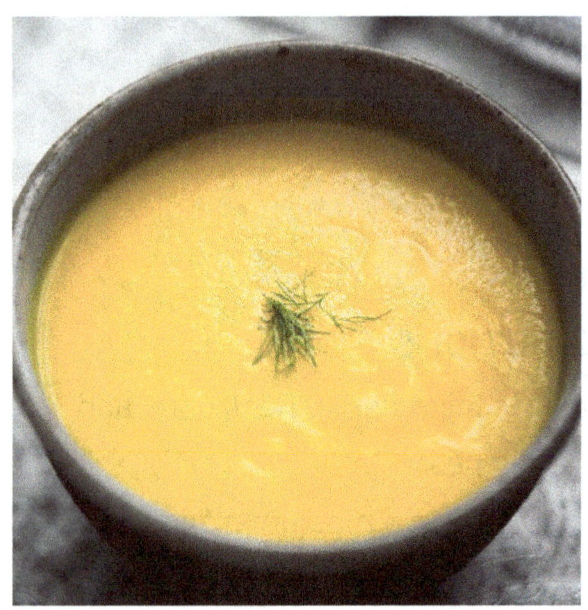

Cook Time: 40 Mins

Serving Size: 4

INGREDIENTS

- 1 tablespoon olive oil
- 1 medium onion, chopped
- 4 large carrots, peeled and chopped
- 1 tablespoon fresh ginger, grated
- 3 cups low-sodium vegetable broth
- 1 cup water
- 1 medium potato, peeled and chopped
- 1 teaspoon turmeric (optional, for added anti-inflammatory benefits)
- 1/2 teaspoon ground cumin
- Salt to taste
- Freshly ground black pepper to taste
- Fresh parsley or cilantro, for garnish (optional)

INSTRUCTIONS

- Sauté: Heat olive oil in a large pot over medium heat. Add chopped onion and sauté for 5 minutes.
- Cook: Add carrots and ginger, cook for 5 minutes. Pour in broth, water, potato, turmeric, and cumin. Bring to a boil, reduce heat, and simmer for 20-25 minutes.
- Blend: Puree the soup with an immersion blender until smooth. Season with salt and pepper.
- Serve: Ladle into bowls and garnish with parsley or cilantro, if desired.

NUTRITIONAL FACTS

- Calories: 120kcal
- Total Fat: 3.5g
- Total Carbohydrates: 20g
- Dietary Fiber: 4g
- Sugars: 7g
- Protein: 2g

BUTTERNUT SQUASH SOUP

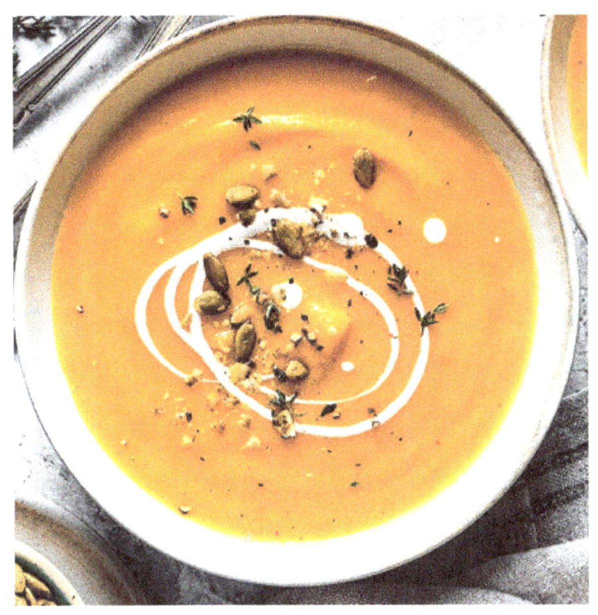

Cook Time: 45 Mins

Serving Size: 4

INGREDIENTS

- 1 medium butternut squash, peeled, seeded, and cubed
- 1 tablespoon olive oil
- 1 medium onion, chopped
- 2 cloves garlic, minced (optional; can be omitted if garlic triggers reflux)
- 1 large carrot, peeled and chopped
- 4 cups low-sodium vegetable broth
- 1 teaspoon fresh ginger, grated
- 1/2 teaspoon ground turmeric
- 1/4 teaspoon ground nutmeg
- Salt and pepper to taste (use sparingly to avoid triggering acid reflux)
- 1/2 cup unsweetened coconut milk (optional, for a creamier texture)

INSTRUCTIONS

- Prepare Squash: Peel, seed, and cube butternut squash.
- Sauté Vegetables: In a pot, heat olive oil over medium. Add onion, sauté 5 minutes. Add garlic (if using), sauté 1-2 minutes.
- Add Ingredients: Add squash, carrot, ginger, turmeric, and nutmeg. Pour in vegetable broth.
- Cook: Bring to a boil, reduce heat, and simmer for 30 minutes until vegetables are tender.
- Blend: Use an immersion blender to puree until smooth. Stir in coconut milk (if using).
- Season and Serve: Add salt and pepper to taste. Garnish with parsley or cilantro if desired.

NUTRITIONAL FACTS

- Calories: 150 kcal | Protein: 2g
- Carbohydrates: 28g | Fiber: 6g
- Sugars: 7g
- Fat: 5g

PUMPKIN SOUP

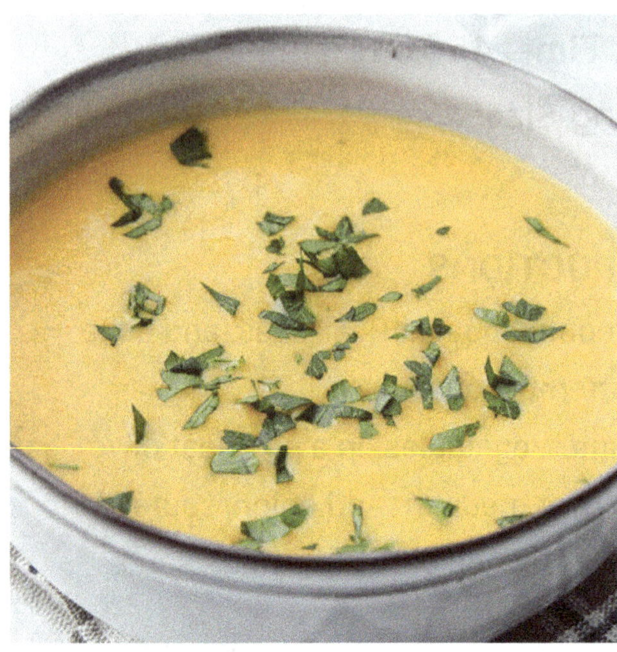

Cook Time: 30 Mins

Serving Size: 4

INGREDIENTS

- 2 cups pumpkin puree
- 1 small onion, chopped
- 2 cloves garlic, minced
- 1 tablespoon olive oil
- 2 cups low-sodium vegetable broth
- 1 teaspoon fresh ginger, grated
- 1/2 teaspoon ground turmeric
- 1/2 teaspoon ground cinnamon
- Salt and pepper to taste
- 1/2 cup unsweetened almond milk (optional)
- Fresh parsley or chives for garnish (optional)

INSTRUCTIONS

- Heat olive oil in a large pot over medium heat. Add chopped onion and minced garlic. Sauté until onions are translucent, about 5 minutes.
- Add pumpkin puree, vegetable broth, grated ginger, turmeric, cinnamon, salt, and pepper to the pot. Stir well to combine.
- Bring the soup to a simmer and let it cook for 15-20 minutes, stirring occasionally.
- If you prefer a creamier consistency, you can blend the soup using an immersion blender or transfer it to a regular blender in batches. If using a regular blender, be sure to let the soup cool slightly before blending.
- Once blended, return the soup to the pot if necessary and stir in unsweetened almond milk for added creaminess (if desired).
- Taste the soup and adjust seasoning if needed.
- Serve hot, garnished with fresh parsley or chives if desired.

GREEN BEAN SOUP

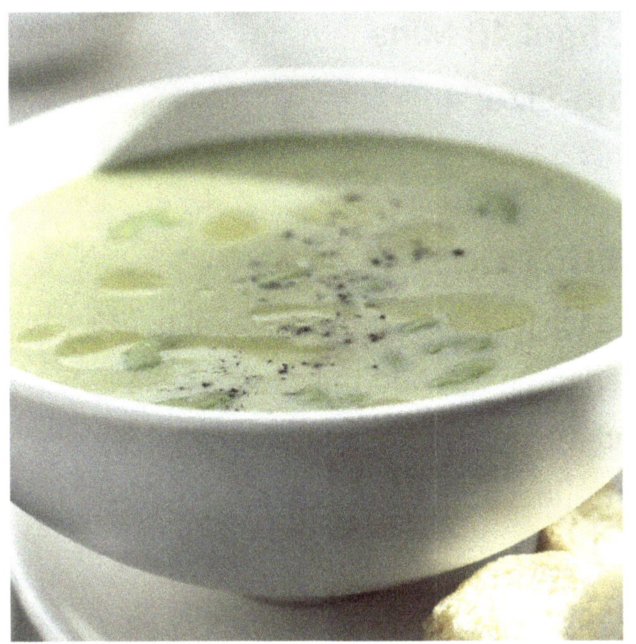

Cook Time: 30 Mins

Serving Size: 4

INSTRUCTIONS

- Heat olive oil in a pot, sauté onion and garlic until soft.
- Add green beans, potato, broth, salt, and pepper.
- Simmer for 20-25 minutes until vegetables are tender.
- Blend until smooth.
- Adjust seasoning if needed.
- Serve hot.

INGREDIENTS

- 1 lb fresh green beans, trimmed and chopped
- 1 medium potato, peeled and diced
- 1 small onion, finely chopped
- 2 cloves garlic, minced
- 4 cups low-sodium chicken or vegetable broth
- 1 tablespoon olive oil
- Salt and pepper to taste
- Optional: 1 teaspoon dried thyme or parsley for added flavor

NUTRITIONAL FACTS

- Calories: 120kcal
- Total Fat: 4g
- Total Carbohydrates: 18g
- Dietary Fiber: 5g
- Sugars: 5g
- Protein: 4g

POTATO LEEK SOUP

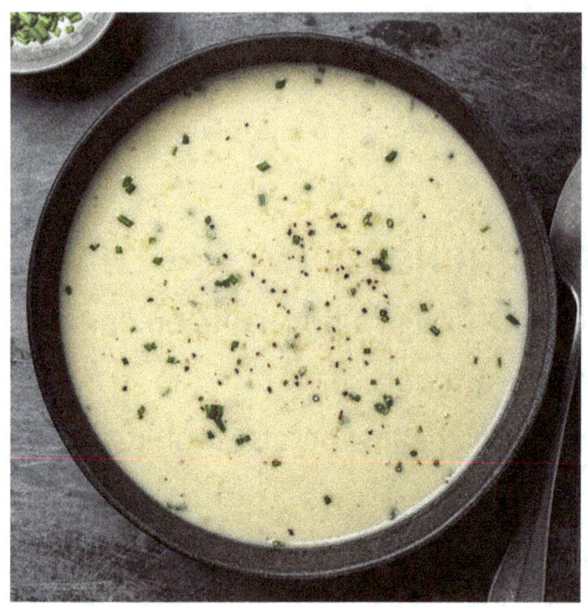

INGREDIENTS

- 4 medium potatoes, peeled and diced
- 2 leeks, white and light green parts only, sliced
- 4 cups low-sodium chicken or vegetable broth
- 1 cup unsweetened almond milk (or other non-dairy milk)
- 2 cloves garlic, minced
- 2 tablespoons olive oil
- Salt and pepper to taste
- Chopped fresh chives for garnish (optional)

NUTRITIONAL FACTS

- Calories: 220 kcal | Total Fat: 7g
- Carbohydrates: 36g | Fiber: 4g
- Sugars: 3g | Protein: 4g

Grill Time: 40 Mins

Serving Size: 4

INSTRUCTIONS

- In a large pot, heat the olive oil over medium heat. Add the sliced leeks and minced garlic. Sauté until softened, about 5 minutes.
- Add the diced potatoes to the pot and pour in the chicken or vegetable broth. Bring to a boil, then reduce the heat to low and simmer for 20-25 minutes, or until the potatoes are tender.
- Using an immersion blender, blend the soup until smooth. Alternatively, you can transfer the soup to a blender in batches and blend until smooth, then return it to the pot.
- Stir in the almond milk and season with salt and pepper to taste. Allow the soup to simmer for an additional 5 minutes.
- Serve hot, garnished with chopped chives if desired.

CUCUMBER SALAD

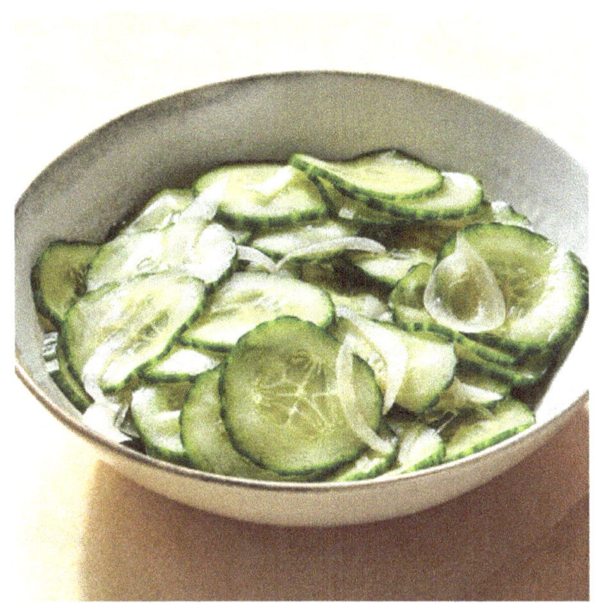

Prep Time: 10 Mins

Serving Size: 4

INGREDIENTS

- 2 large cucumbers, thinly sliced
- 1/4 cup red onion, thinly sliced (optional, can be omitted for those sensitive to onions)
- 2 tablespoons fresh dill, chopped
- 2 tablespoons white wine vinegar (or apple cider vinegar)
- 1 tablespoon olive oil
- 1 teaspoon honey
- Salt to taste
- Freshly ground black pepper to taste

INSTRUCTIONS

- Peel and thinly slice the cucumbers. Place them in a large bowl.
- If using, thinly slice the red onion and add it to the bowl with the cucumbers.
- Add the chopped dill to the bowl.
- In a small bowl, whisk together the white wine vinegar, olive oil, honey, salt, and black pepper until well combined.
- Pour the dressing over the cucumbers and onions (if using), and toss to coat evenly.
- Serve immediately or chill in the refrigerator for a few minutes before serving.

NUTRITIONAL FACTS

- Calories: 60kcal
- Protein: 1g
- Carbohydrates: 7g
- Fat: 3g
- Fiber: 1g
- Sugar: 4g

WATERMELON AND FETA SALAD

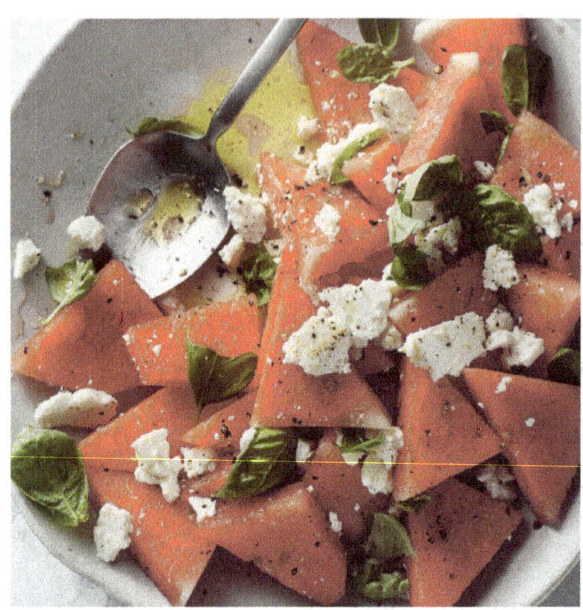

Cook Time: 15 Mins

Serving Size: 4

INSTRUCTIONS

- In a small bowl, whisk together the olive oil, honey, lemon juice, salt, and pepper to make the dressing. Set aside.
- In a large mixing bowl, combine the cubed watermelon, crumbled feta cheese, and chopped mint leaves.
- Drizzle the dressing over the watermelon mixture and gently toss to coat everything evenly.
- Serve immediately or refrigerate until ready to serve.

INGREDIENTS

- 4 cups of cubed seedless watermelon
- 1 cup of crumbled feta cheese (preferably low-fat)
- 1/4 cup of chopped fresh mint leaves
- 2 tablespoons of extra virgin olive oil
- 1 tablespoon of honey
- 1 tablespoon of fresh lemon juice
- Salt and pepper to taste

NUTRITIONAL FACTS

- Calories: 180kcal
- Total Fat: 10g
- Total Carbohydrates: 20g
- Dietary Fiber: 1g
- Sugars: 17g
- Protein: 5g

ROMAINE AND STRAWBERRY SALAD

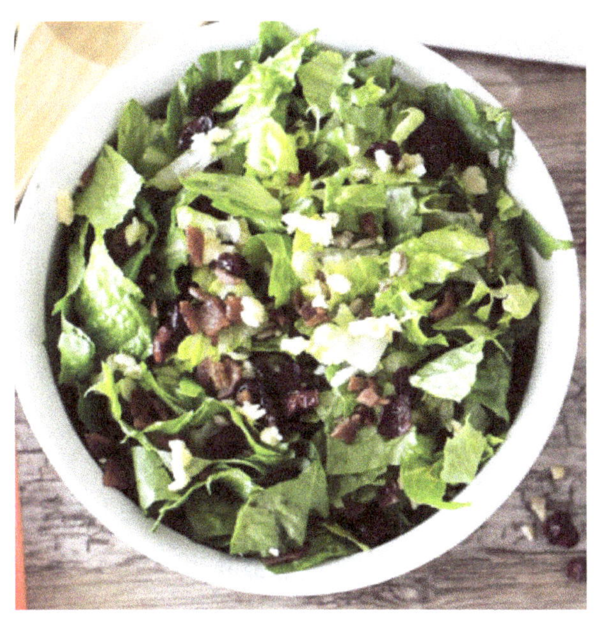

Cook Time: 15 Mins

Serving Size: 4

INSTRUCTIONS

- In a large mixing bowl, combine the chopped romaine lettuce, sliced cucumber, sliced carrots, diced red bell pepper, chopped parsley, and chopped dill.
- Drizzle the extra virgin olive oil and apple cider vinegar over the salad ingredients.
- Season with salt and pepper according to your taste preferences.
- Toss the salad gently until all the ingredients are well combined.
- Optional: Sprinkle the crumbled feta cheese over the salad before serving.
- Serve immediately and enjoy your acid reflux-friendly romaine salad!

INGREDIENTS

- 1 head of romaine lettuce, washed and chopped
- 1 cup sliced cucumber
- 1 cup sliced carrots
- ½ cup diced red bell pepper
- ¼ cup chopped fresh parsley
- ¼ cup chopped fresh dill
- 2 tablespoons extra virgin olive oil
- 2 tablespoons apple cider vinegar
- Salt and pepper to taste
- Optional: ¼ cup crumbled feta cheese (for added flavor, omit if dairy-sensitive)

NUTRITIONAL FACTS

- Calories: 110 kcal
- Fat: 7g
- Carbohydrates: 10g
- Dietary Fiber: 4g
- Sugars: 4g
- Protein: 3g

TURKEY AND RICE CASSEROLE

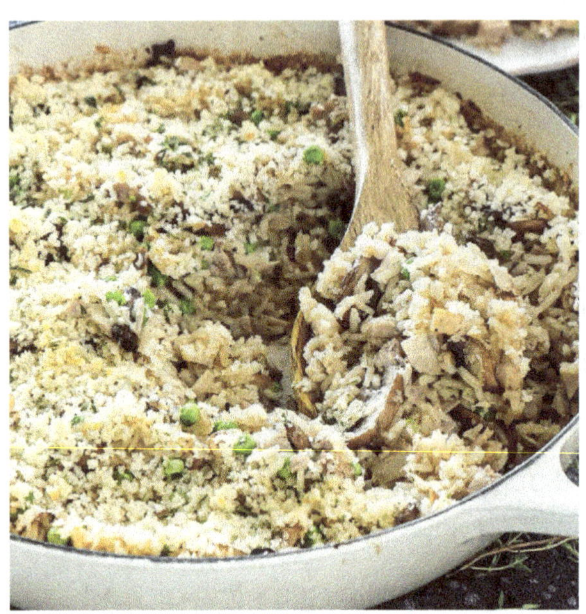

Cook Time: 45 Mins

Serving Size: 6

INSTRUCTIONS

- Preheat oven to 375°F (190°C).
- In a large skillet, cook turkey until no longer pink. Add onion, garlic, carrots, zucchini, and mushrooms. Sauté until tender. Mix in thyme, basil, oregano, turmeric, pepper, and salt.
- In a large bowl, mix turkey-vegetable mixture with uncooked rice. Transfer to a greased 9x13 inch baking dish.
- Pour broth and water over mixture. Cover with foil and bake for 45 minutes.
- If using, remove foil, sprinkle cheese, and bake for an additional 5 minutes.
- Let sit for 5 minutes, garnish with parsley, and serve.

INGREDIENTS

- 1 pound ground turkey breast (lean)
- 1 cup brown rice (uncooked)
- 2 cups low-sodium chicken broth
- 1 cup water
- 1 medium onion, finely chopped
- 2 cloves garlic, minced
- 1 cup carrots, diced
- 1 cup zucchini, diced
- 1 cup mushrooms, sliced
- 1 teaspoon dried thyme
- 1 teaspoon dried basil
- 1 teaspoon dried oregano
- 1 teaspoon ground turmeric
- 1/2 teaspoon ground black pepper
- 1/2 teaspoon salt (optional)
- 1 cup low-fat shredded mozzarella cheese (optional)
- Fresh parsley, chopped (for garnish)

NUTRITIONAL FACTS

- Calories: 310kcal
- Protein: 25g
- Carbohydrates: 40g
- Dietary Fiber: 4g
- Sugars: 3g
- Total Fat: 7g

CHICKEN KABOBS WITH BELL PEPPERS

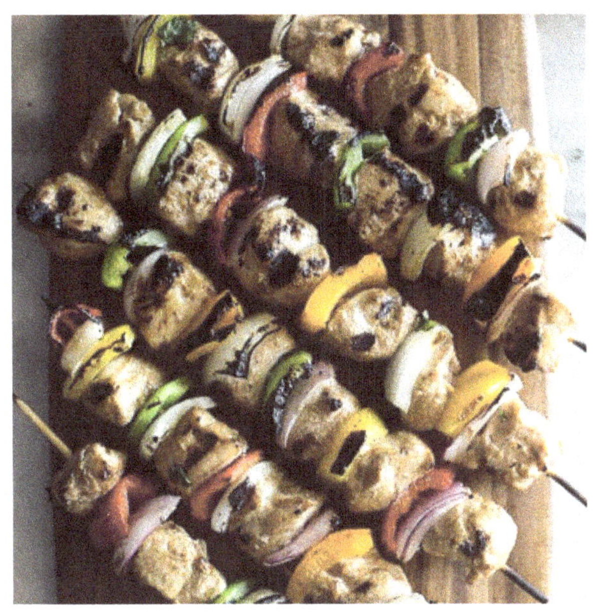

Prep Time: 15 Mins

Marinate Time: 30 Mins (optional)

Cook Time: 15 Mins

Serving Size: 4

INGREDIENTS

- 2 boneless, skinless chicken breasts, cut into 1-inch cubes
- 2 bell peppers (one red, one green), cut into 1-inch pieces
- 1 zucchini, sliced into rounds
- 1 yellow squash, sliced into rounds
- 1 red onion, cut into 1-inch pieces
- 1/4 cup olive oil
- 2 tablespoons lemon juice
- 1 tablespoon dried oregano
- 1 teaspoon garlic powder (optional, as garlic can be a trigger for some people with acid reflux)
- Salt and pepper to taste
- Wooden or metal skewers (if using wooden skewers, soak them in water for 30 minutes prior to use)

INSTRUCTIONS

- **Marinate the Chicken:** In a large bowl, mix olive oil, lemon juice, oregano, garlic powder (if using), salt, and pepper.
- Add the chicken cubes to the bowl and toss to coat. Cover and refrigerate for at least 30 minutes (optional for more flavor).
- **Prepare the Vegetables:** While the chicken is marinating, cut the bell peppers, zucchini, yellow squash, and red onion into 1-inch pieces.
- **Assemble the Kabobs:** Preheat the grill to medium-high heat.
- Thread the chicken and vegetables alternately onto the skewers.
- **Grill the Kabobs:** Place the kabobs on the preheated grill. Cook for about 10-15 minutes, turning occasionally, until the chicken is fully cooked and the vegetables are tender.

NUTRITIONAL FACTS

- Calories: 250kcal
- Protein: 25g
- Total Fat: 12g
- Total Carbohydrates: 10g
- Dietary Fiber: 3g
- Sugars: 5g

INSTRUCTIONS

- Ensure the chicken reaches an internal temperature of 165°F (75°C).
- **Serve:** Remove from the grill and let rest for a few minutes before serving.

ROASTED CHICKEN WITH ROOT VEGETABLES

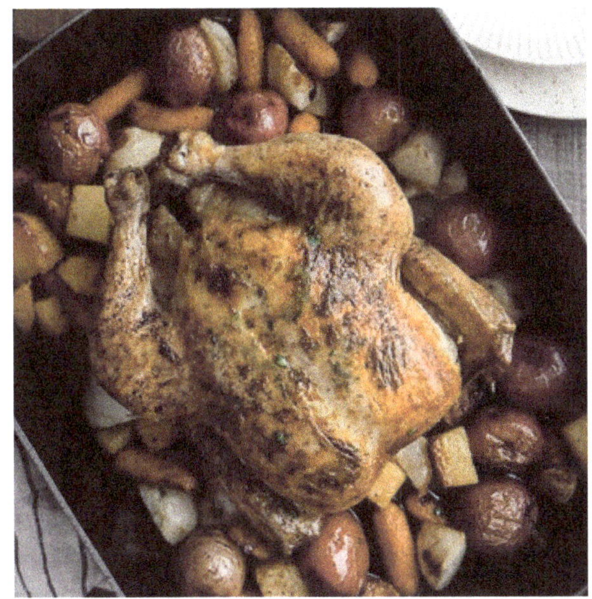

Cook Time: 1 hour 30 Mins

Serving Size: 4

INGREDIENTS

For the Chicken:

- 1 whole chicken (about 4 pounds), giblets removed
- 1 tablespoon olive oil
- 1 teaspoon dried thyme
- 1 teaspoon dried rosemary
- 1 teaspoon dried oregano
- 1 teaspoon salt
- 1/2 teaspoon black pepper
- 1 lemon, quartered
- 4 cloves garlic, smashed
- 1 small onion, quartered

For the Vegetables:

- 3 large carrots, peeled and cut into large chunks
- 2 parsnips, peeled and cut into large chunks

INSTRUCTIONS

- Preheat your oven to 425°F (220°C).
- Rinse the chicken inside and out under cold water, then pat it dry with paper towels.
- Rub the chicken all over with olive oil.
- In a small bowl, mix the thyme, rosemary, oregano, salt, and pepper. Rub this mixture over the chicken, including inside the cavity.
- Place the lemon quarters, smashed garlic cloves, and quartered onion inside the cavity of the chicken.
- Truss the chicken legs with kitchen twine.
- In a large bowl, combine the carrots, parsnips, sweet potatoes, and turnip. Drizzle with olive oil and sprinkle with thyme, rosemary, oregano, salt, and pepper. Toss to coat the vegetables evenly.
- Spread the vegetables in an even layer in a large roasting pan.

INGREDIENTS

- 2 sweet potatoes, peeled and cut into large chunks
- 1 large turnip, peeled and cut into large chunks
- 1 tablespoon olive oil
- 1 teaspoon dried thyme
- 1 teaspoon dried rosemary
- 1 teaspoon dried oregano
- 1/2 teaspoon salt
- 1/4 teaspoon black pepper

NUTRITIONAL FACTS

- Calories: 500kcal
- Protein: 35g
- Carbohydrates: 40g
- Dietary Fiber: 10g
- Sugars: 10g
- Total Fat: 20g

INSTRUCTIONS

- Place the chicken on a rack in the roasting pan, breast side up, over the vegetables.
- Roast in the preheated oven for 1 hour and 20 minutes, or until the chicken reaches an internal temperature of 165°F (74°C) and the juices run clear when the thigh is pierced with a skewer.
- Baste the chicken with its juices halfway through cooking.
- Remove the roasting pan from the oven and tent the chicken with aluminum foil. Let it rest for 10 minutes before carving.
- Stir the vegetables in the pan and return them to the oven for the last 10 minutes if they need additional cooking.
- Carve the chicken and serve with the roasted root vegetables.

HERB-CRUSTED HADDOCK

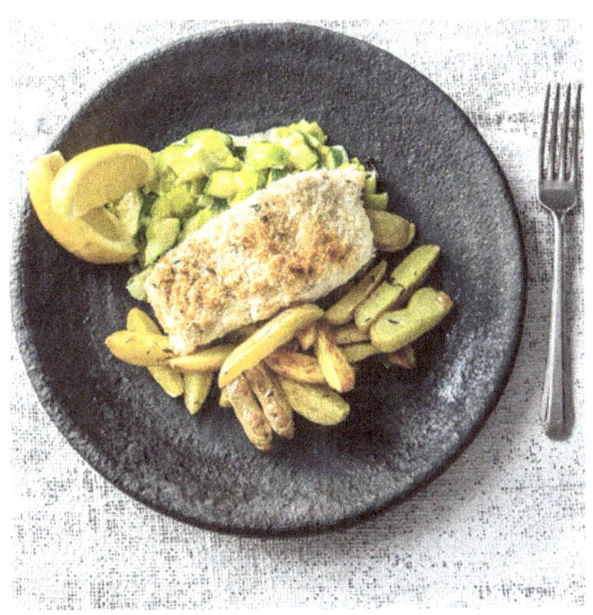

Cook Time: 20 Mins

Serving Size: 4

INSTRUCTIONS

- Preheat the oven: Preheat your oven to 400°F (200°C). Line a baking sheet with parchment paper or lightly spray with cooking spray.
- Prepare the herb crust: In a medium bowl, combine the panko breadcrumbs, parsley, thyme, basil, lemon zest, salt, pepper, and garlic powder. Mix well.
- Coat the haddock: Pat the haddock fillets dry with paper towels. Brush each fillet lightly with olive oil on both sides. Press the fillets into the breadcrumb mixture, coating them evenly.
- Bake the haddock: Place the coated haddock fillets on the prepared baking sheet. Lightly spray the tops with cooking spray to help them brown.
- Cook: Bake in the preheated oven for 15-20 minutes, or until the fish is cooked through and the crust is golden brown.

INGREDIENTS

- 4 haddock fillets (about 6 ounces each)
- 1 cup panko breadcrumbs (whole wheat if available)
- 2 tablespoons fresh parsley, finely chopped
- 2 tablespoons fresh thyme, finely chopped
- 2 tablespoons fresh basil, finely chopped
- 2 tablespoons olive oil
- 1 teaspoon lemon zest
- 1/4 teaspoon salt
- 1/4 teaspoon black pepper
- 1/2 teaspoon garlic powder
- Cooking spray

NUTRITIONAL FACTS

- Calories: 280kcal
- Protein: 30g
- Carbohydrates: 15g
- Dietary Fiber: 2g
- Sugars: 1g
- Fat: 10g

INSTRUCTIONS

- The fish should flake easily with a fork.
- Serve: Serve immediately with a side of steamed vegetables or a simple green salad.

TROUT ALMONDINE

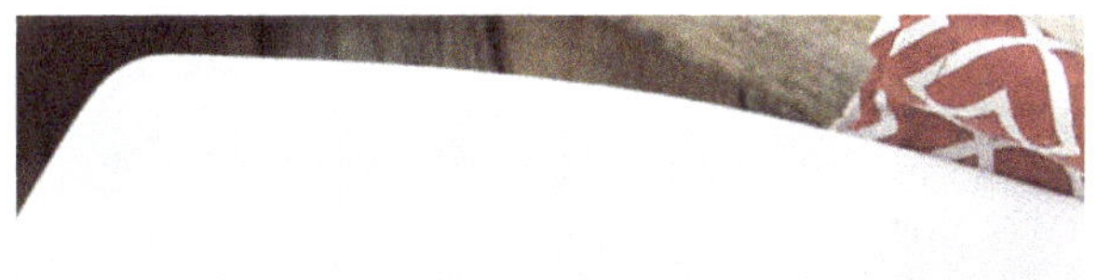

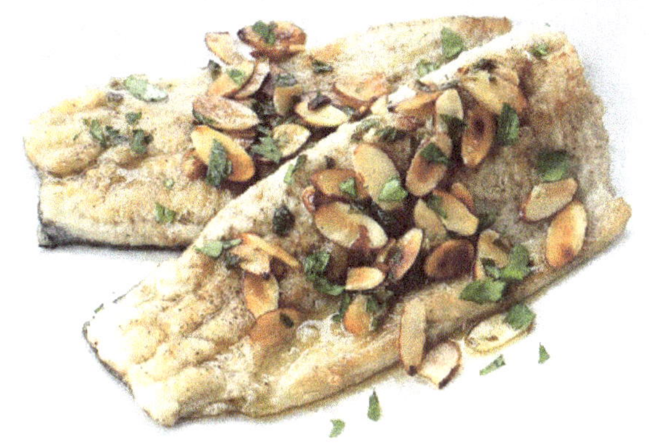

Cook Time: 20 Mins

Serving Size: 4

INGREDIENTS

- 4 trout fillets (about 6 oz each)
- 1/2 cup sliced almonds
- 2 tablespoons unsalted butter (for a lower fat option, use 2 tablespoons olive oil)
- 1 tablespoon olive oil
- 1/2 cup low-sodium chicken broth
- 1 tablespoon fresh lemon juice (optional, depending on tolerance)
- 2 tablespoons fresh parsley, chopped
- 1/4 teaspoon salt
- 1/4 teaspoon black pepper

INSTRUCTIONS

- Pat the trout fillets dry with a paper towel. Season them lightly with salt and black pepper on both sides.
- In a large skillet over medium heat, toast the sliced almonds until they are golden brown. Stir frequently to prevent burning. Once toasted, remove from the skillet and set aside.
- In the same skillet, add 1 tablespoon of olive oil and 1 tablespoon of unsalted butter (or 2 tablespoons olive oil for a lower fat option).
- Once the butter has melted and the oil is hot, add the trout fillets skin-side down. Cook for about 4-5 minutes on each side, or until the fish is opaque and flakes easily with a fork. Remove the fillets from the skillet and keep warm.
- In the same skillet, add the remaining 1 tablespoon of butter (or olive oil if preferred). Once melted, add the low-sodium chicken broth.

NUTRITIONAL FACTS

- Calories: 350kcal
- Protein: 35g
- Carbohydrates: 3g
- Dietary Fiber: 1g
- Sugars: 1g
- Fat: 22g

INSTRUCTIONS

- Stir well, scraping any browned bits from the bottom of the skillet. Let the broth simmer for about 2-3 minutes.
- Add the fresh lemon juice (optional, depending on tolerance) and stir to combine.
- Return the trout fillets to the skillet to warm through for about 1 minute.
- Transfer the trout fillets to serving plates. Pour the sauce over the fillets and sprinkle with the toasted almonds and chopped fresh parsley.
- Serve with a side of steamed vegetables or a light salad.

SHRIMP AND RICE PILAF

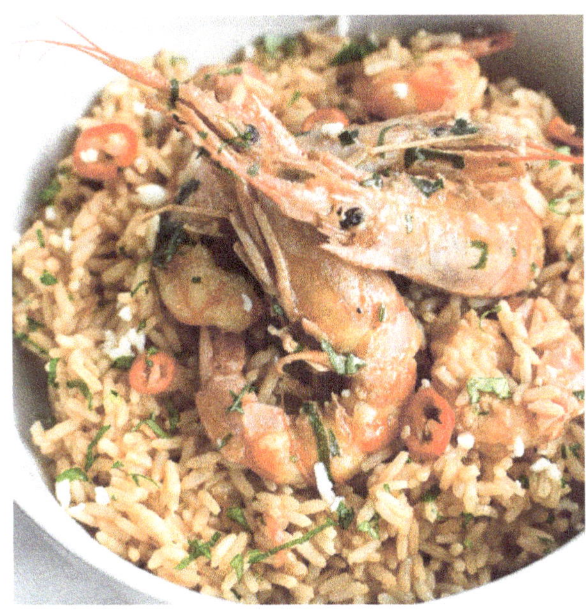

Cook Time: 40 Mins

Serving Size: 4

INGREDIENTS

- 1 cup brown rice
- 2 cups low-sodium chicken or vegetable broth
- 1 tablespoon olive oil
- 1 medium onion, finely chopped
- 2 cloves garlic, minced
- 1 medium carrot, finely diced
- 1 celery stalk, finely diced
- 1 pound large shrimp, peeled and deveined
- 1/2 teaspoon dried thyme
- 1/2 teaspoon dried basil
- 1/2 teaspoon dried oregano
- Salt and pepper to taste (use minimal salt if you're sensitive to it)
- 2 tablespoons fresh parsley, chopped (for garnish)

INSTRUCTIONS

- Boil broth, add rice, cover, and simmer for 30-35 minutes.
- Heat olive oil in a skillet over medium heat. Sauté onion, garlic, carrot, and celery for 5-7 minutes.
- Add shrimp and seasonings to the skillet. Cook until shrimp are pink, about 4-5 minutes. Season with salt and pepper.
- Mix cooked rice with shrimp and vegetables. Heat for 2-3 minutes, garnish with parsley, and serve warm.

NUTRITIONAL FACTS

- Calories: 320
- Protein: 25g
- Total Fat: 6g
- Carbohydrates: 40g
- Dietary Fiber: 4g
- Sugars: 2g

TURKEY MEATLOAF

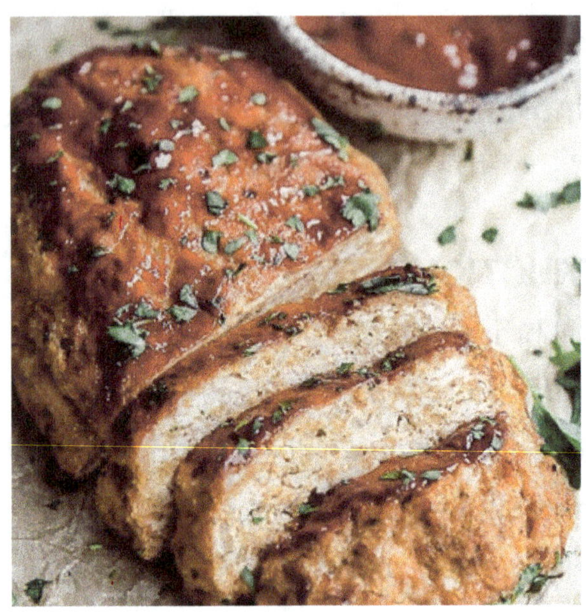

Cook Time: 50 Mins

Serving Size: 4

INGREDIENTS

- 1 pound ground turkey breast
- 1/2 cup rolled oats (gluten-free, if needed)
- 1/2 cup unsweetened applesauce
- 1 small carrot, finely grated
- 1 small zucchini, finely grated
- 1 small onion, finely chopped
- 1 large egg, beaten
- 1 tablespoon fresh parsley, chopped (or 1 teaspoon dried parsley)
- 1 teaspoon dried thyme
- 1/2 teaspoon dried basil
- 1/2 teaspoon dried oregano
- 1/2 teaspoon salt
- 1/4 teaspoon ground black pepper (optional, depending on tolerance)
- 1/4 cup low-sodium chicken broth

INSTRUCTIONS

- Preheat your oven to 375°F (190°C). Lightly grease a loaf pan or line it with parchment paper.
- Grate the carrot and zucchini, and finely chop the onion.
- In a large bowl, combine the ground turkey, rolled oats, applesauce, grated carrot, grated zucchini, chopped onion, beaten egg, parsley, thyme, basil, oregano, salt, and pepper. Mix well until all ingredients are thoroughly combined.
- Add the low-sodium chicken broth to the mixture to keep the meatloaf moist.
- Shape the mixture into a loaf shape and place it in the prepared loaf pan.
- Bake in the preheated oven for about 50 minutes or until the internal temperature reaches 165°F (74°C).
- Allow the meatloaf to rest for 10 minutes before slicing and serving.

PRAWN COCKTAIL WITH AVOCADO

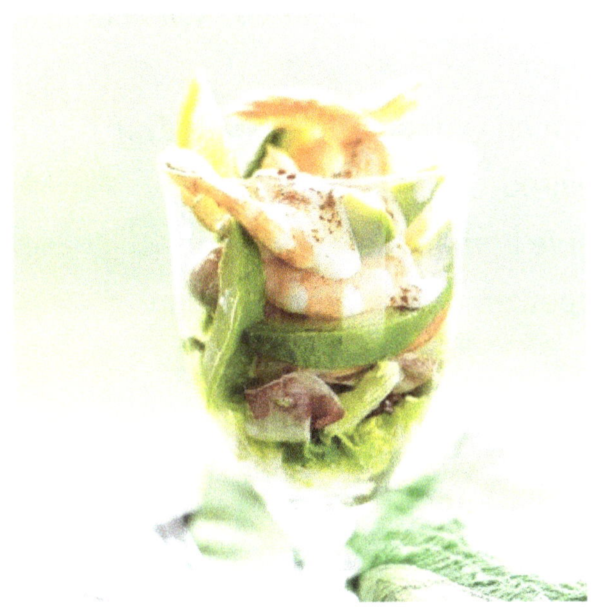

Cook Time: 5 Mins

Serving Size: 4

INGREDIENTS

For the Prawns:

- 1 lb (450g) cooked prawns, peeled and deveined
- 1 tablespoon olive oil
- 1 teaspoon lemon juice (use in moderation)
- Salt to taste
- Freshly ground black pepper to taste (optional, use sparingly)

For the Avocado Mixture:

- 2 ripe avocados, diced
- 1 small cucumber, diced
- 1/4 cup red onion, finely chopped (optional, use sparingly)
- 1 tablespoon fresh parsley, chopped
- 1 tablespoon olive oil

INSTRUCTIONS

- In a bowl, mix the cooked prawns with olive oil, lemon juice, salt, and pepper.
- Set aside to marinate briefly while preparing the avocado mixture.
- In a large bowl, combine diced avocados, cucumber, red onion (if using), and parsley.
- Drizzle with olive oil and lemon juice.
- Season with salt to taste.
- Gently mix until well combined, being careful not to mash the avocado too much.
- In a small bowl, whisk together Greek yogurt, ketchup, lemon juice, Worcestershire sauce (if using), and paprika.
- Mix until smooth and well combined.
- In serving glasses or bowls, layer the avocado mixture at the bottom.
- Top with a portion of the marinated prawns.

INGREDIENTS

- 1 teaspoon lemon juice (use in moderation)
- Salt to taste

For the Cocktail Sauce:

- 1/2 cup Greek yogurt
- 2 tablespoons ketchup (low-sugar)
- 1 teaspoon lemon juice (use in moderation)
- 1/2 teaspoon Worcestershire sauce (optional, use sparingly)
- 1/4 teaspoon paprika

INSTRUCTIONS

- Drizzle with the prepared cocktail sauce.
- Garnish with additional parsley if desired.
- Serve immediately as a light appetizer or a refreshing salad.

NUTRITIONAL FACTS

- Calories: 290
- Protein: 23g
- Total Fat: 20g
- Saturated Fat: 3g
- Cholesterol: 180mg
- Sodium: 500mg
- Total Carbohydrates: 10g
- Dietary Fiber: 5g
- Sugars: 3g

MILLET PILAF

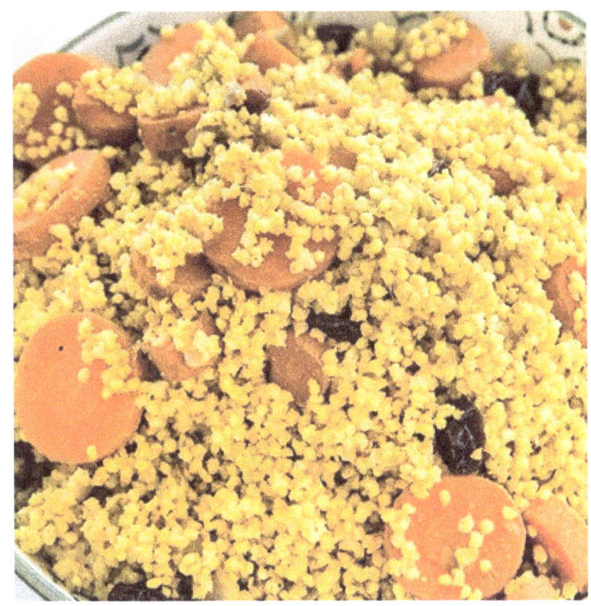

Cook Time: 45 Mins

Serving Size: 4

INGREDIENTS

- 1 cup millet
- 2 cups water
- 1 tablespoon olive oil
- 1 teaspoon cumin seeds
- 1 medium carrot, diced
- 1 small zucchini, diced
- 1/2 cup green peas (fresh or frozen)
- 1/4 teaspoon turmeric powder
- 1/4 teaspoon ground coriander
- 1/2 teaspoon salt (or to taste)
- 2 tablespoons chopped fresh parsley or cilantro
- 1 lemon, cut into wedges (optional for serving)

INSTRUCTIONS

- Rinse the millet under cold water. In a medium saucepan, bring 2 cups of water to a boil. Add the rinsed millet, reduce the heat to low, cover, and simmer for about 20 minutes or until the water is absorbed and the millet is tender. Remove from heat and let it sit, covered, for an additional 5 minutes. Fluff with a fork.
- While the millet is cooking, heat the olive oil in a large skillet over medium heat. Add the cumin seeds and cook for about 1 minute until they are fragrant.
- Add the diced carrot, zucchini, and green peas to the skillet. Sauté for about 5-7 minutes until the vegetables are tender.
- Add the turmeric powder, ground coriander, and salt to the skillet. Stir well to combine and cook for another 2 minutes.

NUTRITIONAL FACTS

- Calories: 220kcal
- Protein: 6g
- Carbohydrates: 36g
- Dietary Fiber: 5g
- Sugars: 3g
- Fat: 6g

INSTRUCTIONS

- Add the cooked millet to the skillet with the vegetables. Stir well to combine and cook for an additional 3-5 minutes, allowing the flavors to meld together.
- Remove from heat and stir in the chopped fresh parsley or cilantro. Serve the pilaf warm, with lemon wedges on the side if desired.

TEFF PANCAKES

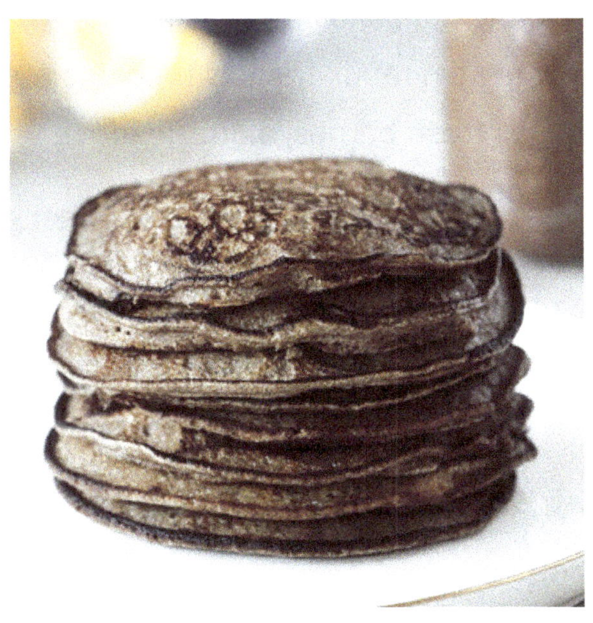

Cook Time: 15 Mins

Serving Size: 2

INSTRUCTIONS

- In a large bowl, whisk together the Teff flour, baking powder, baking soda, salt, and ground flaxseed.
- In another bowl, mix the applesauce, almond milk, melted coconut oil, vanilla extract, and maple syrup (if using) until well combined.
- Pour the wet ingredients into the dry ingredients. Stir until just combined, being careful not to overmix. The batter should be slightly thick and lumpy.
- Preheat a non-stick skillet or griddle over medium heat. Lightly grease with a small amount of coconut oil.
- Pour 1/4 cup of batter onto the skillet for each pancake. Cook until bubbles form on the surface and the edges look set, about 2-3 minutes. Flip and cook for another 2-3 minutes, or until golden brown.

INGREDIENTS

- 1 cup teff flour
- 1 teaspoon baking powder
- 1/2 teaspoon baking soda
- 1/4 teaspoon salt
- 1 tablespoon ground flaxseed
- 1/2 cup unsweetened applesauce
- 1 cup unsweetened almond milk (or other non-dairy milk)
- 1 tablespoon coconut oil, melted (plus extra for greasing the pan)
- 1 teaspoon vanilla extract
- 1 tablespoon maple syrup (optional, for added sweetness)

NUTRITIONAL FACTS

- Calories: 200kcal
- Total Fat: 6g
- Total Carbohydrates: 32g
- Dietary Fiber: 5g
- Sugars: 6g
- Protein: 5g

INSTRUCTIONS

- Serve the pancakes warm with your favorite acid reflux-friendly toppings, such as fresh berries, a drizzle of pure maple syrup, or a dollop of non-dairy yogurt.

BULGUR WHEAT TABBOULEH

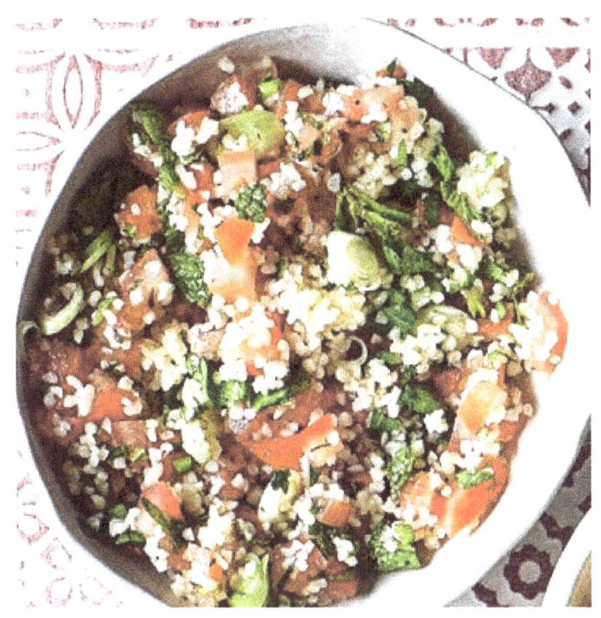

Cook Time: 30 Mins

Serving Size: 4

INSTRUCTIONS

- Place the bulgur wheat in a large bowl.
- Pour the boiling water over the bulgur and cover the bowl.
- Let it sit for about 15-20 minutes until the bulgur is tender and has absorbed the water.
- Fluff the bulgur with a fork.
- While the bulgur is soaking, finely chop the parsley, mint, cucumber, tomatoes, and green onions.
- In a large mixing bowl, combine the chopped parsley, mint, cucumber, tomatoes, and green onions.
- Once the bulgur is ready, add it to the bowl with the chopped vegetables.
- Add the extra virgin olive oil and freshly squeezed lemon juice to the mixture.

INGREDIENTS

- 1 cup bulgur wheat
- 1 1/2 cups boiling water
- 1 cup finely chopped fresh parsley
- 1/2 cup finely chopped fresh mint
- 1 cup diced cucumber
- 1 cup diced tomatoes (optional, or substitute with yellow tomatoes if red tomatoes cause issues)
- 1/4 cup finely chopped green onions (white parts omitted if they cause issues)
- 1/4 cup extra virgin olive oil
- 1/4 cup freshly squeezed lemon juice (reduce to taste if lemon is a trigger)
- Salt to taste
- Freshly ground black pepper to taste

NUTRITIONAL FACTS

- Calories: 180 kcal
- Protein: 4g
- Carbohydrates: 26g
- Dietary Fiber: 6g
- Sugars: 2g
- Total Fat: 8g

INSTRUCTIONS

- Season with salt and freshly ground black pepper to taste.
- Stir the ingredients until well combined.
- Refrigerate the tabbouleh for at least 30 minutes before serving to allow the flavors to meld.

VANILLA BEAN PANNA COTTA

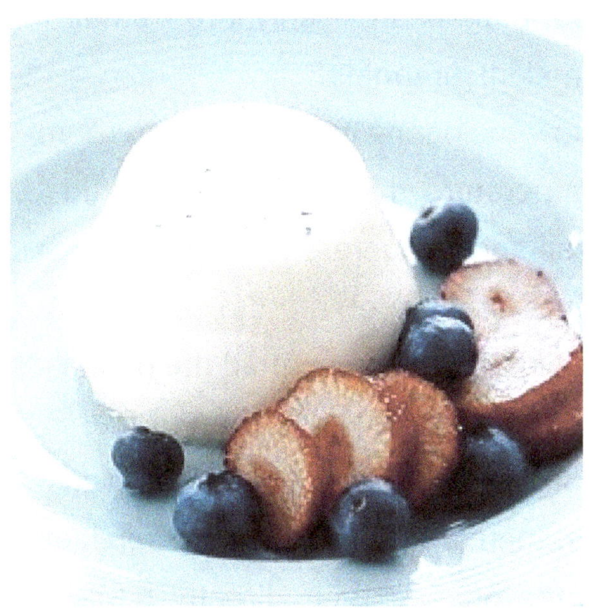

Cooking: 5 minutes

Chilling: 4 hours

Serving Size: 4

INGREDIENTS

- 1 cup whole milk
- 1 cup heavy cream
- 1 vanilla bean
- 1/4 cup honey (instead of sugar, to reduce acid reflux risk)
- 1 packet (about 2 1/4 tsp) unflavored gelatin
- 3 tbsp cold water

INSTRUCTIONS

- Slice the vanilla bean lengthwise and scrape out the seeds with the back of a knife.
- In a small bowl, sprinkle the gelatin over the cold water and let it sit for about 5 minutes until it softens and blooms.
- In a saucepan, combine the milk, cream, honey, vanilla bean seeds, and the pod.
- Heat the mixture over medium heat until it just starts to simmer. Do not let it boil.
- Remove the saucepan from the heat. Discard the vanilla bean pod.
- Add the bloomed gelatin to the hot milk mixture and stir until completely dissolved.
- For a smoother panna cotta, strain the mixture through a fine sieve into a large measuring cup or bowl with a spout.

NUTRITIONAL FACTS

- Calories: 220kcal
- Protein: 4g
- Total Fat: 15g
- Saturated Fat: 9g
- Carbohydrates: 20g
- Sugars: 19g
- Fiber: 0g

INSTRUCTIONS

- Pour the mixture evenly into 4 small ramekins or molds.
- Allow the panna cotta to cool to room temperature, then cover with plastic wrap and refrigerate for at least 4 hours, or until set.
- To serve, you can unmold the panna cotta by dipping the bottom of the molds in hot water for a few seconds and then inverting them onto serving plates, or serve them directly in the ramekins.

MANDARIN & ALMOND CAKE

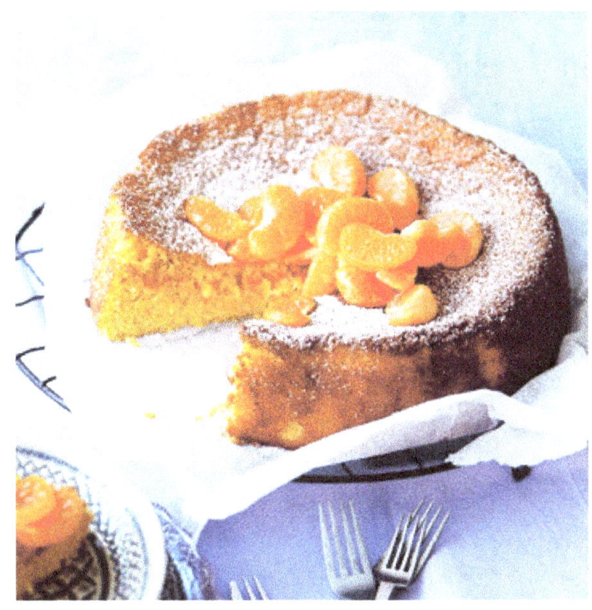

Cook Time: 40 Mins

Serving Size: 8

INGREDIENTS

- 2 cups almond flour
- 1 teaspoon baking powder
- 1/4 teaspoon baking soda
- 1/4 teaspoon salt
- 3 large eggs
- 1/2 cup honey
- 1/4 cup unsweetened applesauce
- 1 teaspoon vanilla extract
- 1/2 cup mandarin juice (from about 4-5 mandarins)
- 1 tablespoon mandarin zest (optional, avoid if sensitive to citrus peels)

INSTRUCTIONS

- Preheat your oven to 350°F (175°C). Grease and line a 9-inch round cake pan with parchment paper.
- Prepare Dry Ingredients: In a medium bowl, whisk together the almond flour, baking powder, baking soda, and salt.
- Mix Wet Ingredients: In a large bowl, beat the eggs until frothy. Add the honey, applesauce, vanilla extract, mandarin juice, and mandarin zest (if using). Mix well.
- Combine Ingredients: Gradually add the dry ingredients to the wet ingredients, stirring until just combined.
- Pour and Bake: Pour the batter into the prepared cake pan and spread evenly. Bake for 35-40 minutes, or until a toothpick inserted into the center comes out clean.

NUTRITIONAL FACTS

- Calories: 220
- Total Fat: 14g
- Total Carbohydrates: 18g
- Dietary Fiber: 3g
- Sugars: 12g
- Protein: 7g

INSTRUCTIONS

- Cool: Allow the cake to cool in the pan for about 10 minutes, then transfer it to a wire rack to cool completely.

CHERRY ALMOND CLAFOUTIS

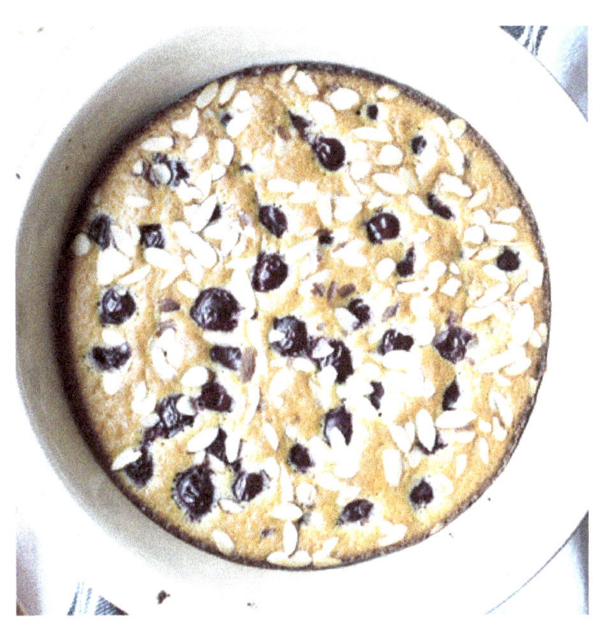

Cook Time: 40 Mins

Serving Size: 6

INGREDIENTS

- 2 cups fresh cherries, pitted
- 3 large eggs
- 1/2 cup almond flour
- 1/2 cup oat milk (or any non-dairy milk)
- 1/4 cup maple syrup or honey
- 1 tsp vanilla extract
- 1/4 tsp almond extract
- 1/4 tsp salt
- 1/4 tsp ground cinnamon
- Powdered sugar (optional, for dusting)

INSTRUCTIONS

- **Preheat Oven:** Preheat your oven to 350°F (175°C). Lightly grease a 9-inch pie dish or baking dish.
- **Prepare Cherries:** Spread the pitted cherries evenly in the bottom of the prepared dish.
- **Mix Batter:** In a mixing bowl, whisk together the eggs, almond flour, oat milk, maple syrup (or honey), vanilla extract, almond extract, salt, and ground cinnamon until smooth.
- **Combine and Pour:** Pour the batter over the cherries in the dish.
- **Bake:** Bake in the preheated oven for 35-40 minutes, or until the clafoutis is puffed and golden, and a toothpick inserted into the center comes out clean.
- **Cool and Serve:** Allow to cool slightly. Dust with powdered sugar if desired before serving.

NUTRITIONAL FACTS

- Calories: 160 | Protein: 5g
- Fat: 8g | Carbohydrates: 19g
- Fiber: 2g | Sugar: 14g

NOTE:

CHOCOLATE COCONUT BREAD

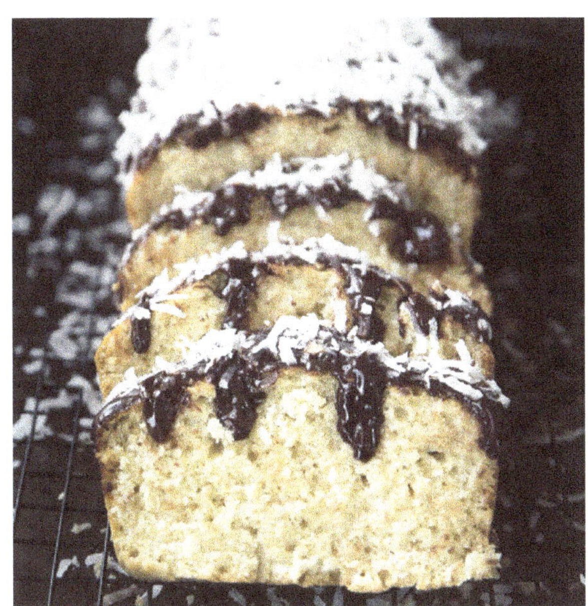

INGREDIENTS

Dry Ingredients:

- 1 ½ cups whole wheat flour
- 1 teaspoon baking powder
- ½ teaspoon baking soda
- ¼ teaspoon salt
- ½ cup unsweetened cocoa powder

Wet Ingredients:

- ½ cup coconut oil, melted
- ½ cup unsweetened applesauce
- ½ cup honey or maple syrup
- 2 large eggs
- 1 teaspoon vanilla extract
- 1 cup unsweetened almond milk

Add-ins:

- ½ cup unsweetened shredded coconut
- ¼ cup dark chocolate chips (optional)

Baking: 45 minutes

Serving Size: 10

INSTRUCTIONS

- **Preheat the oven:** to 350°F (175°C). Grease a 9x5-inch loaf pan or line it with parchment paper.
- **Combine dry ingredients:** In a large mixing bowl, whisk together the whole wheat flour, baking powder, baking soda, salt, and cocoa powder until well combined.
- **Mix wet ingredients:** In another bowl, whisk together the melted coconut oil, applesauce, honey or maple syrup, eggs, vanilla extract, and almond milk until smooth.
- **Combine wet and dry ingredients:** Pour the wet ingredients into the dry ingredients and mix until just combined. Be careful not to overmix.
- **Fold in add-ins:** Gently fold in the shredded coconut and dark chocolate chips (if using).
- **Transfer to the loaf pan:** Pour the batter into the prepared loaf pan and spread it evenly.

NUTRITIONAL FACTS

- Calories: 220
- Total Fat: 12g
- Total Carbohydrates: 27g
- Dietary Fiber: 3g
- Sugars: 12g
- Protein: 4g

INSTRUCTIONS

- **Bake:** Place the loaf pan in the preheated oven and bake for 45 minutes, or until a toothpick inserted into the center comes out clean.
- **Cool:** Allow the bread to cool in the pan for 10 minutes, then transfer it to a wire rack to cool completely before slicing.

MANGO NICE CREAM

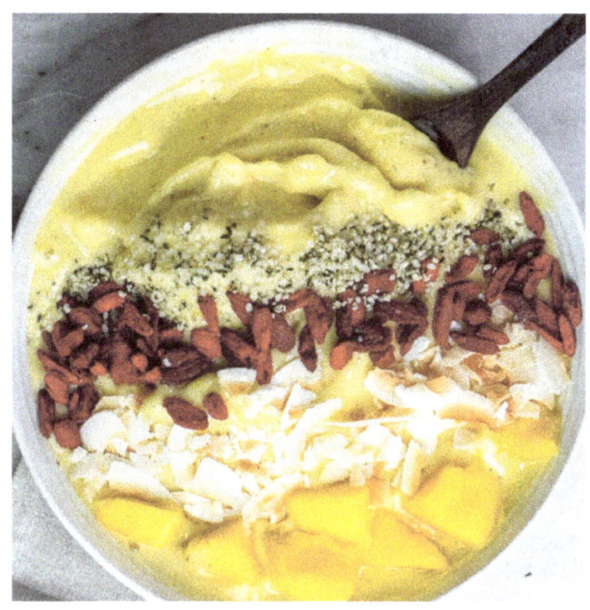

**Freezing Time: 4 hours
(if using fresh mangoes)
Serving Size: 4**

INSTRUCTIONS

- Freeze Fruit: Peel, slice, and freeze mangoes and banana for 4 hours.
- Blend: Combine frozen mango, banana, coconut milk, and vanilla in a blender. Blend until smooth. Add more coconut milk if needed.
- Sweeten: Add honey or maple syrup if desired and blend again.
- Serve or Freeze: Serve immediately for soft-serve or freeze for 1-2 hours for a firmer texture.

INGREDIENTS

- 3 cups of frozen mango chunks (about 3 medium-sized mangoes)
- 1 ripe banana, sliced and frozen
- 1/2 cup unsweetened coconut milk (or any non-dairy milk)
- 1 teaspoon pure vanilla extract
- 1-2 tablespoons of honey or maple syrup (optional, to taste)

NUTRITIONAL FACTS

- Calories: 110
- Total Fat: 1g
- Total Carbohydrates: 28g
- Dietary Fiber: 3g
- Sugars: 24g
- Protein: 1g

GINGER TEA

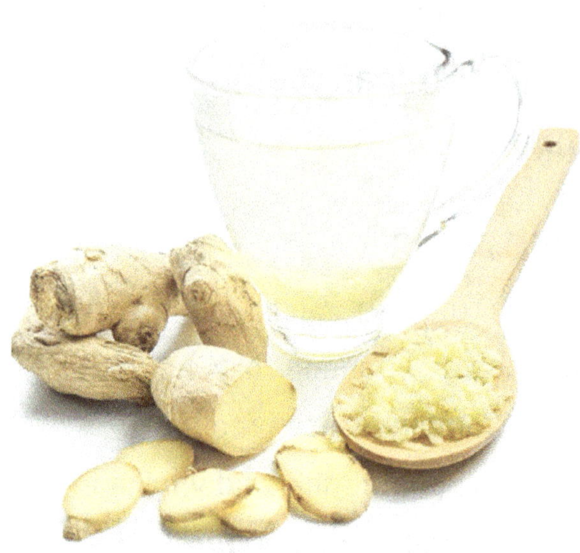

Cook Time: 15 Mins

Serving Size: 1

INGREDIENTS

- 1-inch piece of fresh ginger root
- 2 cups of water
- 1 tablespoon of honey (optional)
- 1 tablespoon of lemon juice (optional)

NUTRITIONAL FACTS

- Calories: 10 (without honey and lemon)
- Total Fat: 0g
- Sodium: 0mg
- Total Carbohydrates: 2g
- Dietary Fiber: 0g
- Sugars: 0g (without honey)
- Protein: 0g

INSTRUCTIONS

- Prepare the Ginger: Peel the ginger root and slice it thinly.
- Boil the Water: In a small pot, bring 2 cups of water to a boil.
- Add Ginger: Add the sliced ginger to the boiling water.
- Simmer: Reduce the heat and let the ginger simmer in the water for 10 minutes.
- Strain: Remove the pot from the heat and strain the tea to remove the ginger slices.
- Add Honey and Lemon (Optional): If desired, stir in honey and lemon juice to taste.
- Serve: Pour the tea into a cup and enjoy warm.

CUCUMBER WATER

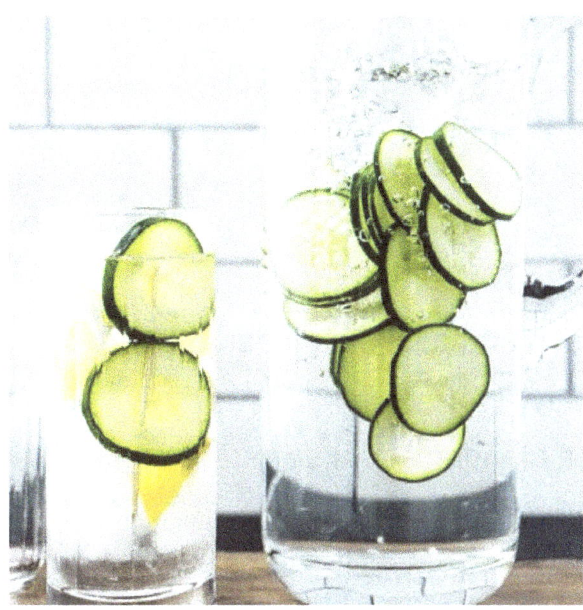

Cook Time: 10 Mins

Serving Size: 4

INGREDIENTS

- 1 medium cucumber
- 4 cups of water
- 1 small lemon (optional)
- A few fresh mint leaves (optional)

NUTRITIONAL FACTS

- Calories: 7
- Carbohydrates: 2g
- Protein: 0g
- Fat: 0g
- Fiber: 0g
- Sugar: 0g

INSTRUCTIONS

- Wash the cucumber and ginger thoroughly.
- Slice the cucumber into thin rounds.
- Peel and thinly slice the ginger.
- If using, slice the lemon into thin rounds.
- In a large pitcher, add the cucumber slices, ginger slices, lemon slices, and mint leaves.
- Pour in the water.
- Stir gently and refrigerate for at least 1 hour to let the flavors infuse.
- Serve chilled, adding ice cubes if desired.

ALOE VERA-GINGER JUICE

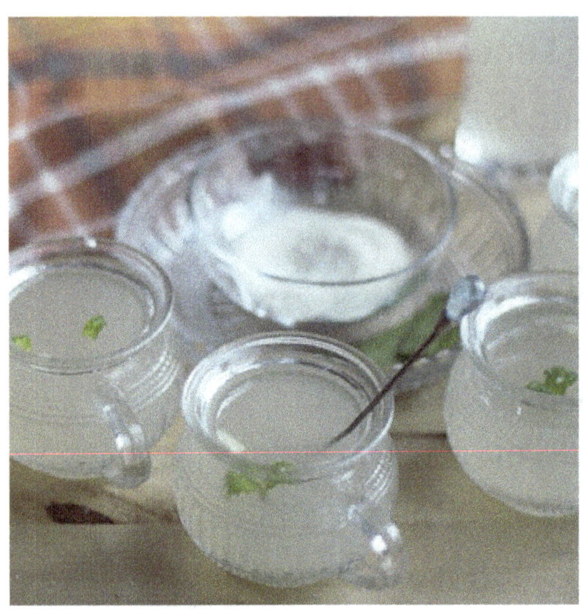

Cook Time: 10 Mins

Serving Size: 2

INGREDIENTS

- 1/4 cup aloe vera gel (store-bought or extracted from aloe vera leaves)
- 1 small piece of fresh ginger (about 1 inch)
- 1 apple (peeled and cored)
- 1 cup water
- Honey to taste (optional)

INSTRUCTIONS

- Wash and peel the ginger. Grate it finely.
- In a blender, add aloe vera gel, grated ginger, apple, and water.
- Blend until smooth.
- Strain the mixture through a fine-mesh sieve or cheesecloth into a jug to remove pulp.
- Add honey to taste if desired and stir well.
- Serve chilled.

NUTRITIONAL FACTS

- Calories: 60
- Protein: 0.5g
- Carbohydrates: 15g
- Fiber: 1.5g
- Sugars: 12g
- Fat: 0g

CARROT-APPLE JUICE

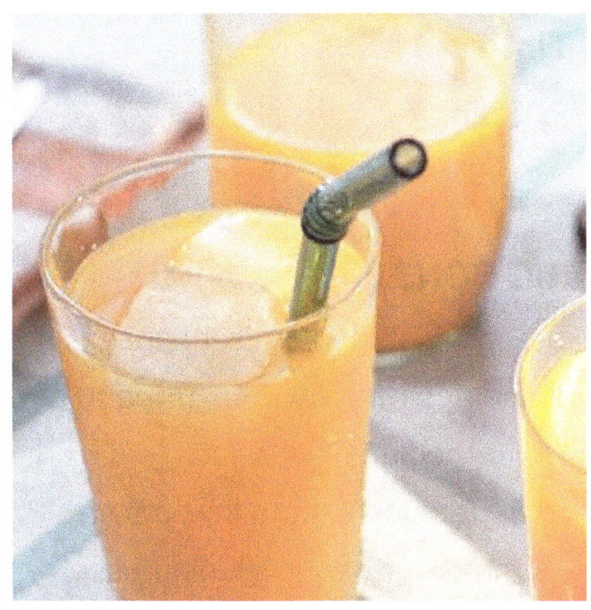

Cook Time: 10 Mins

Serving Size: 2

INSTRUCTIONS

- Wash and peel the carrots and ginger. Cut them into chunks.
- Add carrot chunks, apple, ginger, and water to a blender.
- Blend until smooth.
- Strain the mixture through a fine-mesh sieve or cheesecloth into a jug to remove pulp.
- Serve immediately.

INGREDIENTS

- 3 medium carrots
- 2 apples (peeled and cored)
- 1/2 inch fresh ginger
- 1 cup water

NUTRITIONAL FACTS

- Calories: 90
- Protein: 1g
- Carbohydrates: 22g
- Fiber: 4g
- Sugars: 17g
- Fat: 0g

RICE MILK PUDDING

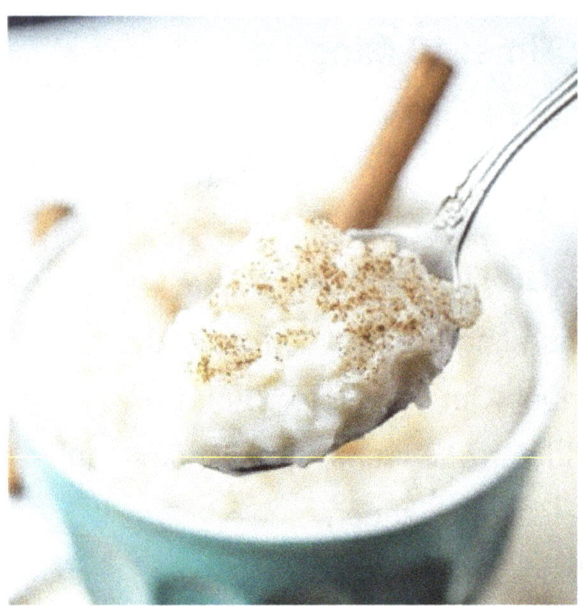

Cook Time: 20 Mins

Serving Size: 4

INSTRUCTIONS

- Cook Rice: In a medium saucepan, combine rice milk and rice. Bring to a boil over medium-high heat.
- Simmer: Reduce heat to low, cover, and simmer for about 15 minutes, or until the rice is tender.
- Sweeten: Stir in the maple syrup or honey, vanilla extract, ground cinnamon, and salt. Cook for an additional 5 minutes, stirring frequently, until the pudding thickens.
- Serve: Serve warm or chilled. Store any leftovers in the refrigerator for up to 3 days.

INGREDIENTS

- 2 cups rice milk (from recipe above)
- 1/4 cup white rice
- 1/4 cup maple syrup or honey
- 1 teaspoon vanilla extract
- 1/2 teaspoon ground cinnamon
- Pinch of salt

NUTRITIONAL FACTS

- Calories: 120
- Protein: 2g
- Carbohydrates: 26g
- Fat: 1g
- Fiber: 1g
- Sugars: 12g

NOTE:

NOTE:

NOTE:

NOTE:

NOTE:

NOTE: